Natural Healing and Medical Research

Emmanuil Ioannis Misodoulakis

Copyright:

Author: [Evexiandros]
Editor: [Emmanouil Ioannis Misodoulakis]
Copyright © [Emmanouil Ioannis Misodoulakis]

First Published, February 2022

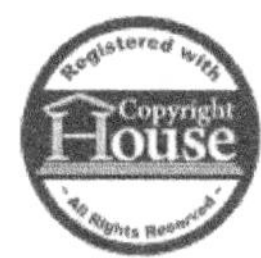

Table of Contents:

About the Author:

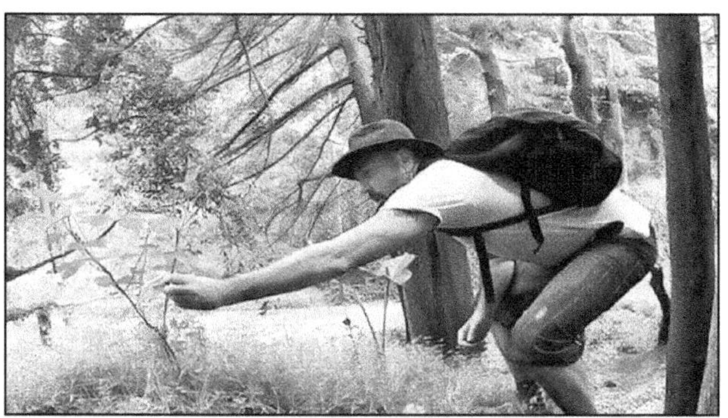

My name is Emmanuel, I'm an author, documentary filmmaker, certified yoga instructor, and a certified healer in Thai Massage & USUI Reiki, but besides that, I'm a natural medicine researcher. My real passion is the search for wellness and spirituality. My author's pen name is "Evexiandros", I chose that name as according to the Ancient Greeks; names should be created by the way you live your life. I travel around the world and I explore traditional medicine secrets, alternative treatments, folk healing practices, superfoods, athletic activities, meditation techniques, and philosophy pathways. I'm seeking healing in every corner of this planet. Evexiandros in Greek means Men of Wellness, much like my website: (the wellness seeker).

*"Let food be thy medicine,
and let medicine be thy food"*
Hippocrates

Introduction:

Natural Healing and Medical Research...

Wellness is a state of physical, mental, and spiritual balance and is the only path to bliss. Scientists today starting to understand how wild animals use plant medicines to prevent diseases. With Zoopharmacognosy, many exotic plant species were used to treat health conditions by many healers. Herbs and Medicinal parts of the plants are used by many ethnic groups around the world. In this book, I investigate the secrets of traditional medicine and determine whether or not these secrets are supported by clinical studies.

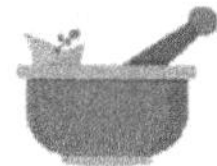

Traditional medicine secrets, natural treatments, folk healing practices, superfoods, physical activities for well-being, longevity, and of course medical research. I will share holistic and powerful effective remedies for living a better life. Treatments for many medical problems such as upper and lower respiratory diseases like allergies and asthma, stomach problems like gastritis, and acid reflux, tooth disorders, viral, bacterial, and fungal diseases, cardiovascular diseases, mental health concerns like anxiety, and so on.

Please Consider Leaving a Review:

Writing a book takes a lot of time and effort. If you enjoyed this book and feel that you gained knowledge regarding your overall wellness, please consider leaving a review, just a line or two is enough. I will appreciate it very much, as reviews are very important for independent authors like me.

Thank You.

LONGEVITY SECRETS

I was always curious about the secrets to longevity and how some people can live to 100 or even more. My Grandfather died at 97 years old after all. For sure everyone wants to live a long life, however, having a happy life is what I consider to be most vital. For achieving this, you will need some life changes. So, let's discover together the secrets of the longevity of these long lived-people, and try to do the same. We will research the mythological part and of course the scientific part of longevity.

Top Places where People Live the Longest:

Here are the top places where people live the longest. Let's study what is the secrets of the people who reached longevity in those places. Nutrition, exercise, and no stress are for sure some of their secrets.

Acciaroli – Italy

Acciaroli is located in southern Italy and believe it or not, more than one in ten people live beyond 100 years. Another great thing is the low rates of heart disease and Alzheimer's in those super-agers. According to studies from the University of California, San Diego School of Medicine, and University of Rome La Sapienz those long-living people have very good blood circulation (low levels of adrenomedullin hormone) and their bodies can absorb all the nutrients. It is not clear why Acciaroli is so special. It's probably a combination of the Mediterranean diet and exercise.

Sardinia – Italy

Sardinia is one of the largest islands of the Mediterranean Sea, with a lot of history, traditions, and places to see. But besides that, Sardinia is also one of the five Blue Zones of longevity. Studies showed that eating habits, genes, and social life perhaps are the secrets to the Sardinian population's long life.

Okinawa – Japan

Japanese people have the highest life expectancy, 90 for women and 84 for men. Okinawa is the largest of the Ryukyu Islands and it belongs to the five world blue zones. It is also known as the "land of the immortals". But more than that, Okinawans have low rates of cancer, heart disease, stroke, and diabetes. Some said that if an Okinawan moves to a new place it's going to lose the super-ager powers. This leads me to the conclusion that Okinawans' longevity is not only about genetics, but has to do more with environmental, and lifestyle factors.

Loma Linda – California

Another place that is famous for longevity and that is also a blue zone is Loma Linda of San Bernardino in California. The citizens of Loma Linda are Adventists and are ten times more likely to live to one hundred than any other American. This city focused on health and wellness. No drinking, no smoking, no caffeine. Lacto-Ovo vegetarianism and regular exercise may also be some of the longevity secrets of Loma Linda residents.

Nicoya Peninsula – Costa Rica

Another Blue Zone region is the Nicoya Peninsula in Costa Rica. Nicoyans eat meat only a few times a week, they avoid processed food and eat a lot of vegetables. Physical activity is also a part of daily life. Another explanation for the longevity of that region is that the drinking water in the Nicoya Peninsula is rich in minerals and especially calcium. Finally, because of the sun the vitamin (hormone) D protects Nicoyans from strokes, diabetes, and heart disease.

Ikaria – Greece

Ikaria in Greece is part of the Cyclades group and also a blue zone region. People on this island live long and healthy lives and more than 30% of the island residents live over the age of 90. People here have little to no stress. Locals tell "we are in Ikaria, the island where you don't need to hurry". The Mediterranean diet is also important. Another factor is the radioactive hot spring healing spas that were famous from ancient times. Radiation Hormesis is an old and effective healing treatment.

Andorra – Between France and Spain

Andorra it's the 16th smallest country in the world, surrounded by France and Spain. It's a famous tourist spot for wellness and holistic health. With an average life expectancy of 83 years, Andorra ranks as the eighth-highest country in the world. Because of the Mountains (some of which are over 2000 meters high), people are active and the air is cleaner. Andorra has also the Tour De France, the world's best cycle race.

Vilcabamba – Ecuador

Vilcabamba is a village in the southern part of Ecuador that is situated in a highland valley. It is also known as the sacred valley by the Incas or the valley of longevity. Some old people of Vilcabamba are over 100 years old, and some it's said to have reached the age of 120. The place has attracted scientists who study the people of Vilcabamba for a long time now. Climate, water that is clean and packed with minerals, an organic diet, and a life full of activity are the secrets of Vilcabamban's longevity.

Macau – China

I visited Macau long ago, and I have to say that it is a beautiful clean place. Macau has its own money, is totally separate from China, and yes, is among the cities with the highest life expectancy on the planet. What makes people live longer in Macau? Wealth is for sure the first, a clean diet with fresh vegetables is the second, and lastly, free healthcare vouchers for all citizens and high-quality medical care round out the list.

Abkhazia – Georgia

Abkhazia is located on the eastern coast of the Black Sea in northwestern Georgia. Here the people are known for their incredible longevity and lifespans. Many travelers are amazed by the longevity and good health of this Caucasian race. There is also a legend, about an Abkhasian man named Shirali Muslimov, that died 168 years old.

San Marino:

San Marino is the 5th smallest country in the world, surrounded by Italy's Le Marche and Emilia-Romagna regions. The average life expectancy is 83 years. People are less stressed, and one of San Marino's best kept secrets is Mediterranean cuisine made with local herbs and vegetables.

Hunza Valley – Diet and Longevity Secrets:

Long ago, during the 70s, National Geographic magazine ran an extensive series of articles about long-lived people around the world. Hunza People have known for their amazing longevity and health. The life expectancy of the average Westerner is about 70 years. Hunza people reach the venerable age of one hundred. Some people believe that Hunza's life expectancy is a myth, while others say it is true. Some even say that the Hunza Valley was the basis for Shangri La in the book Lost Horizons. Who can tell what is true and what is a lie? Others agree to the fact that the Hunza people are descendants of Alexander the Great and yes, they could very well be Greek! According to the local Burusho legend, the village was founded by the army of Alexander the Great. There is anyway a connection between the Hunza and the neighboring Kalash people of Pakistan, who also claim to have Alexandrian ancestry. Some people think that Hunza's longevity is a hoax because Hunza people do not keep records and there is no birth certificate to prove their age. Dr. John Clark, who spent 20 months there, writing his Book – The Lost Kingdom of the Himalayas, said that the Hunza people also suffered from malaria, dysentery, and many other diseases. However, it is a fact that all reports of the Hunza, mention that the elderly population is fit, full of vitality, and virtually free from diseases like cancer.

Some researchers have called the Hunza the happiest people on Earth. So, what are the Hunza diet secrets that allow these people to live such long lives while remaining healthy?

Hunza Diet and Longevity Secrets:

Nutrition:
'You are what you eat.' Hunzas diet was "Prescribed" by the ancient Greek doctor Hippocrates. All they eat are fresh and raw. Grains, fruits, vegetables, yogurt, fresh meat, and nuts.

Apricots:
Hunzas eat large amounts of apricots that are rich in Amygdalin. According to studies, apricots are the secret behind the absence of cancer tumors.

Hunzas are not Stressed:
Tension and stress are unknown to Hunzas.

Hunza Valley:
Since it supplies them with clean mountain air to breathe and fresh water for drinking and bathing, the Valley is one of the best kept secrets of the Hunza people.

Hunza People are Active:
Another secret is the exercise which normally is done outdoors to take advantage of the pure mountain air.

Fasting:
Hunzas fast for several days in the spring.

Hwangchil Dendro-panax:

Dendropanax Morbiferus, often known as the "elixir of life," is a cure for all diseases! Dendro (Δέντρο) in Greek language means "tree" and Panax (Πανάκεια) means "drug for all diseases." Some people state that is five times stronger than Ginseng. Genghis Khan used to drink a cup of Hwangchil before the battles as a tonic. The juice of this tree is gold. Koreans used the juice to clean their gold jewelry. The healing effects of Hwangchil Dendropanax were so incredible that they were recorded as an elixir by Qin Shi Huang (King of the state of Qin who conquered all other warring states and united China in 221 BC). A drop of Hwangchil juice on your tongue can naturally make you reach the condition of Suseung Hwagang (water up, fire down principle) a fundamental dynamic of energy that is maintained by the balance of hot and cold. Today a form of Hwangchil has become a new health supplement. There was a general understanding that Hwangchil Dendropanax ordinarily grows in the wild only in Korea (Jeju Island), but today we found out that there are Hwangchil trees in Japan as well! Like ginseng root, Hwangchil is an adaptogenic herb with antimicrobial action and antioxidant effects that works as an Anti-Aging Elixir and promotes brain activity.

Why Did Hwangchil Tree Disappear from History?
The use of Hwangchil was forbidden even in the Korean imperial court of the royal palace. It was so precious in China that all of Hwangchil from Korea was demanded as a tribute. It caused such hardship for the Koreans, that they cut all the trees down with axes.

Radiation Hormesis and Longevity:

It all started when I wanted to research more about the beautiful Greek island of Ikaria, which is famous mainly for one thing, LONGEVITY. I study everything about the food and the habits of those old-timers, and it was then, that I found out all about the Radioactive Hot Springs of Ikaria Island. The residents of Ikaria Island in Greece live long, healthy lives, and as I mentioned before more than 30% of the island residents live over the age of 90. The springs of Ikaria are still popular and most of the old-timers still visit them monthly. The radioactive hot springs baths have been popular since ancient times. Some famous ancient springs of Ikaria were buried 300 meters east of where Therma is today.

Are Low Dose Radioactive Hot Springs Safe?

So, after reading and researching more about the radioactive hot springs, I had a question: If radiation is as dangerous as many people believe, why does one-third of Ikaria's population live past the age of 90? Radiation Hormesis is an old but extremely effective healing treatment. Did you know that in the 20th century after the discovery of radioactivity in 1896 by French physicist and Nobel Prize winner Antoine Henri Becquerel, radium was hailed as a panacea and used as a new treatment to cure many ailments? Products containing radium were everywhere. In cosmetics, in heating pads and suppositories, in clocks and watches, in water, and so on…

Radium is still in household products today, and in small amounts is considered not harmful by the governments. Brazil nuts contain naturally small amounts of radium and are about 1000 times higher than any other common food. The radium content in Brazil nuts is not dangerous on a relative basis. Today Radiation therapy uses high-energy radiation to shrink tumors and kill cancer cells. Unfortunately, high radiation can damage DNA and cause more problems.

The Anti-Aging Benefits of Fasting:

The discipline of fasting dates to ancient times. This detoxification method was thought to have healing properties by the ancient Greeks and Pythagoras, Hippocrates, Socrates, Plato, and Aristotle were also staunch supporters of fasting. There are many famous quotes about the discipline of fasting like: "If you can control what you eat, you can control all other aspects of your life." -Mike Dolce. "Hunger is the first element of self-discipline. If you can control what you eat and drink, you can control everything else." -DR. UMAR FARUQ ABD- ALLAH.

3 Days Fasting Regenerates the Entire Immune System:

Although fasting diets according to some nutritionists are unhealthy, many new studies have shown that during fasting the body forces the stem cells to produce new white blood cells, which fight infection. Prolonged fasting helps the body to use the stocks of glucose. During each cycle of fasting, this depletion of leukocytes induces changes that activate the stem cells to regenerate new cells of the immune system. Dr. Longo says "When we are hungry, our immune system tries to save energy, and in order to do that, our body recycling many of the immune cells that are not needed, particularly those that may have been damaged".

Intermittent Fasting Slows Aging:

It doesn't matter what diet you do, Keto, paleo, vegan, or raw food diet, intermittent fasting is good for everybody. We all know by now that intermittent fasting has a lot of benefits: Encourages weight loss, reduces insulin resistance and inflammation in the body, improves blood sugar, and helps to heal the gut. But what about aging? From the beginning of humanity, we were trying to find ways to stay younger, but what if there is a simple way to stay young? Fasting is common in many religions around the world. It is in our DNA, don't forget that our ancestors often experienced extended periods of hunger. Yes, intermittent fasting is ancient, and it is the oldest and most powerful dietary plan. While you fast, your body naturally cleanses itself through a process called autophagy. Autophagy is derived from two Greek words: auto (self) and phagy (eating). So, it simply means self-eating. A new fasting study that was released on September 6, 2018, provides evidence for the theory that elevation during fasting has anti-aging effects. Another Harvard study published on October 26, 2017, in Cell Metabolism shows how intermittent fasting may increase lifespan. Finally, a previous study also showed how intermittent fasting can slow aging. I do mostly the 14/10 and 16/8 intermittent fasting methods and work fine. It keeps me lean, boosts my metabolism, improves my sleep, boosts my immune system, and hopefully, it improves longevity.

Sauna Anti-Aging Benefits:

S aunas and steam rooms are my favorite way to relax after a hard workout. When we think about saunas our mind goes directly to Scandinavia in places like Sweden and Finland but in reality, the history of saunas and steam rooms is elder. Mayans used sweathouses for religious ceremonies and healing purposes. Byzantine Greek, Roman (300 BC), and Turkish steam baths "hammams" were very famous in the ancient world. Finally, Japanese Onsen and Korean Jimjilbang bathhouses were famous in Asia. In short, the anti-aging health benefits offered by a sauna were known to all from ancient times.

Can you Sweat out Toxins?

Sweating is a natural body process. The purpose of sweating is to prevent overheating. But what about toxins? Can you sweat out toxins? You will hear many times from some so-called experts that heavy sweating is not an effective method of ridding your body's toxins and that sweating releases traces of toxins as is composed of 99 percent water and a tiny percent of salt, urea, and some proteins and carbohydrates. Fortunately, they are wrong. The use of a sauna helps to detox our lymphatic system. The lymphatic system allows the toxins to exit via sweat. Our skin is our third kidney. How do I know that? Look at all of those that have kidney failure or any other kidney disease. The first thing that the body does is to flush toxins out from the skin and that's the reason that patients with kidney problems have rashes. Simply put, a skin rash or itching indicates that the kidneys are removing waste from the bloodstream. Heat improves circulation and helps the lymph system to move and excrete toxins.

The Secret Detoxification of Sauna and Niacin:

Want to flash toxins even faster and achieve longevity? Here is a secret, and it's called Dr. Yu's Detoxification Protocol. Dr. Yu's Detoxification Protocol is a combination of Niacin (also known as B3), exercise, sauna, and activated charcoal. A dose of 50 to 250 mg of Niacin helps to crack open the cell wall and take out toxins from the fat cells. Together with exercise and sauna causes lipolysis and detoxification. Take the niacin dose and start exercise (this increases the lymphatic circulation) for 20 to 30 minutes. Finally, stay in the sauna for 15 to 20 minutes and also consume 500 mg of activated charcoal. Niacin supplements are made in the lab from synthetic organic compounds and are water-soluble, so it is not stored in the body. According to studies and many experts including Dr. Rhonda Patrick, sitting in a sauna, or steam room for 20 to 30 minutes can stimulate the natural production of HGH (human growth hormone). Also, sauna lowers all-cause mortality as well, as a 50% lower cardiovascular disease-related mortality.

Sauna Heat-Stress Proteins:

Heat stress increases the production of HSPs (Heat Shock Proteins). HSPs help our immune system to stabilize our proteins, prevent Parkinson's, Dementia, and Alzheimer's diseases. Another benefit of heat stress is the activation of the FOXO3 Gene. According to studies, FOXO3 activity is very important as it affects lifespan and healthy aging and is the best way to repair our DNA.

Other Sauna Benefits:

Regulates Body Temperature: The purpose of sweating is to prevent overheating. ***Sweating Kill Viruses:*** Bacteria cannot survive in temperatures above 98.6 degrees Fahrenheit. ***Sweat Cleans the Skin:*** It improves your skin's elasticity and tone. ***It Helps Fight Sickness:*** Sweating can help your body to get rid of your sickness.

It Improves Blood Flow: Improve blood circulation naturally by using a sauna. ***Can Relief Pain:*** Saunas are ideal for people who suffer from chronic pain.

It Helps with Weight Loss: The use of a sauna is perfect for burning visceral fat (the fat surrounding the organs).

Saunas Boost the Immune System: The heat generated in the sauna will boost your immune system immediately.

It Helps to Recover from Workouts: Relief of muscle tension leads to quicker recovery between workouts.

It Relieves Stress: Yes, saunas are a great way to relieve stress.

Anti-Aging Molecules:

If you do a search for "longevity" online, you will find articles about all these different nutrients, including vitamins A, E, D, C, and K, collagen, omega-3 fatty acids, polyphenols, carotenoids, flavonoids, prebiotics, probiotics, minerals like magnesium and zinc, and finally creatine, taurine, glutamine, and other amino acids. This is fine, but I'd like to delve a little deeper into the science and mainly into Anti-aging molecules like NAD, NAC, Glutathione, Niacin, NRF2, DHEA, GCG, and FOXO3, which, in my opinion, are more important for longevity.

Niacin = Niagen = NAD: According to studies, NAD is one the most important anti-aging molecules and reverses aging from inside your body as it repairs damaged DNA. NIAGEN (nicotinamide riboside) is a member of the vitamin B3 family. NAD is a derivative of nicotinamide, which nicotinamide is a derivative of the common niacin (vitamin B3). Nicotinamide does not cause skin flushing associated with niacin and is also converted faster to NAD in the body. Unfortunately, NAD+ levels decline with age, which can reduce lifespan, cause DNA damage, inflammation, and mitochondrial dysfunction. So how can I increase my NAD naturally? A fasting and calorie restriction diet has been shown to increase NAD+ levels. Niacin supplements are also a solution.

Glutathione: Glutathione is the most important antioxidant in the body. It's all you need to stay young, healthy and prevent any disease. It is found in large quantities in the liver. Glutathione plays a crucial role in detoxification as it enables our liver to cleanse from harmful chemicals. This amino acid can be synthesized in the body from other amino acids like L-glutamic acid, L-cysteine, and glycine. Unfortunately, some experts say that GSH supplements are not working. So, what to do instant? Try to raise your glutathione levels by taking large amounts of the amino acids of which glutathione is synthesized, like whey protein and cysteine, or other antioxidants, like vitamin C, Silymarin (milk thistle), and lipoic acid. Raw whey protein, cold processed Non-Denatured, from grass-fed pasture-raised Cows is one of the best ways to raise glutathione levels. Raw organic whey was subjected to less heat treatment. For that reason, whey keeps all of the amino acids and other potent nutrients and substances that can improve our immune system. I bought an Australian raw organic whey and it was the best whey I ever taste. If you have lactose intolerance, try A2 milk whey protein. Milk produced by A1 cows produces some bad side effects, especially for people with lactose intolerance. So if you have lactose problems, try to get A2 milk whey protein.

N-Acetyl Cysteine – NAC: As I mentioned before L-cysteine (along with glycine and glutamine) helps your body to produce glutathione, the most important antioxidant for our body and one of the best anti-aging molecules. So, the NAC supplement is a very good option if you want to stay young and healthy. NAC can fight free radicals even without glutathione, and studies have shown that it helps with many other health problems like Depression, OCD, Addictions, Testosterone Imbalance, Autism, Respiratory Diseases, ADHD, Alzheimer's, Liver disease, and Parkinson's disease. Some foods contain L-Cysteine in small doses like salmon, chicken, turkey, cheese, spinach, tomatoes, cabbage, beets, sunflower seeds, yogurt, asparagus, eggs, and legumes. NAC supplement, in general, is not good to use for a long time. It is better to use it as a tool for detoxification periods.

DHEA – Dehydroepiandrosterone: DHEA is actually a steroid pro-hormone that is produced by our adrenal glands, but men also secrete it from their testes. Dehydroepiandrosterone (DHEA) helps to produce hormones like testosterone and estrogen. Unfortunately, DHEA production is getting dramatically low with age. In the United States, DHEA supplements were banned by the FDA in 1985 and allowed again in 1994. Many people take DHEA supplements for health benefits and to prevent aging. DHEA helps with longevity, builds lean muscle mass, improves bone density, lowers inflammation, lowers diabetes risk, protects against depression, controls cholesterol levels, fights fatigue, promotes heart health, and can even improve libido. The bad news is that many studies showed that high doses of DHEA may increase the risk of cancers that are affected by hormones. There are no food sources for DHEA. Wild yams and soybeans contain substances that are similar to DHEA and are used to create a "bio-identical" DHEA. Most Bio-identical hormones are molecules made from plant materials that have the same structure as hormones made by the body. Ok, so what we can do to avoid the side effects of Bioidentical hormones replacement? To boost your DHEA levels naturally, you have to first, eat more healthy fats and limit sugar and carbs, as elevated insulin blocks DHEA production. Second, heal your adrenal glands by fasting or dry fasting. Third, exercise daily and eliminate stress.

Epigallocatechin Gallate – EGCG: Tea, in general, is rich in polyphenols, but green tea has more polyphenols, including flavonoids, and an antioxidant called catechin (EGCG). It is the most powerful green tea molecule. What foods except green tea contain EGCG? Peaches, berries, pecans, pistachios, hazelnuts, plums, avocados, pears, apples, kiwis, white tea, black tea, and oolong tea also contain small amounts of EGCG. Research showed that EGCG can help with aging and many other health problems such as heart disease, brain disorders, obesity, diabetes, and certain malignancies. Do I need EGCG supplementation? Some experts believe that EGCG supplements should come with a warning as studies showed that higher doses of EGCG can cause liver damage. A single cup of green tea contains about 80 to 100 mg of EGCG, so just drink green tea.

KEAP1 – NRF1-NRF2: Nrf2/nrf1 genes are 2 very important proteins and together with the enzyme Keap1 regulate over 600 genes. Helping the body with detoxification and cell defense gene expression. The Keap1-Nrf2 pathway also protects the body from cancers, Alzheimer's disease, Parkinson's disease, multiple sclerosis, diabetes, hormonal imbalance, autism, atherosclerosis, rheumatoid arthritis, and so on. There are many foods and herbs that can help with the activation of the antioxidant Nrf2. Sulforaphane is one of the best ways to active Keap1-nrf2. Broccoli or broccoli sprouts are rich in sulforaphane. Resveratrol is a natural phenol and a phytoalexin found in many foods like grapes, blueberries, cranberries, peanuts, pistachios, red and white wine, and cocoa. Resveratrol may prevent inflammation and oxidative stress by activating Nrf2 and SIRT1. Curcumin is a yellow polyphenol compound found in turmeric and is also a very good Keap1-nrf2 activator. Catechins as I mentioned before are phytonutrients called flavanols found in tea, especially green tea, apples, apricots, peaches, berries, and cocoa. As flavonoids, catechins activate Nrf2. Some people try an easier way to activate NRF2 like supplementation with Protandim. Several studies have shown that Protandim can potently activate the Nrf2-driven gene. Protandim contains five herbal ingredients, ashwagandha, green tea extract, bacopa extract, milk thistle-silymarin, and curcumin. Unfortunately, some studies on human subjects showed that Protandim did not increase antioxidant activity and has a lot of side effects.

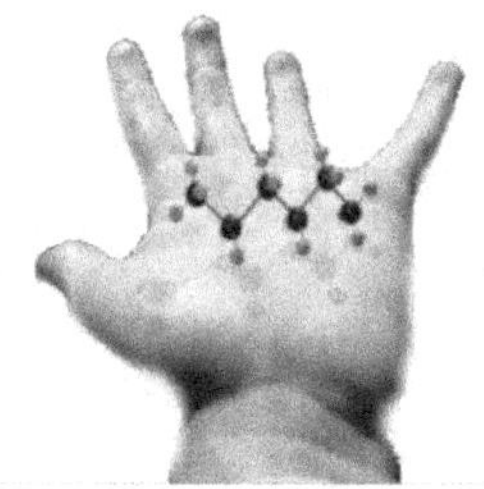

FOXO3: The FoxO proteins family (FOXO1, FOXO3, FOXO4, and FOXO6) are involved in apoptosis energy cell cycle regulation and metabolic processes. The FoxOs activity might hold promise in cancer therapy. FOXO activity also affects lifespan and healthy aging and is promising in repairing DNA damage.

Activate FOXO3 Gene:

Caloric Restriction and Intermittent Fasting:
Yes, both caloric restriction and intermittent fasting induce activation of (FoxO) proteins.

Exercise:
Working out is one of the best ways to activate foxo3 Gene.

Sauna:
Ronda Patrick and many other scientists explain how sauna increased the expression of heat shock proteins and activates the foxo3 gene.

FOOD SOURCES OF FOXO3:
Vitamin D, Mushrooms, Green tea polyphenols like EGCG, Selenium, Baicalein from Chinese skullcap, and Quercetin found in onions and apples can also increase FOXO3. Alpha-lipoic acid foods like broccoli, spinach, and organic red meat.

NUTRITION AND HERBAL MEDICINES

Explore the world of herbal medicine. Herbal medicine has been utilized to treat illness by several civilizations since the dawn of time. Investigate the advantages of fruits and veggies. Nutrition is a crucial aspect of health and development. Healthy eating habits extend lifespan and decrease the risk of serious health problems. With healthy eating, we become more energized and happier.

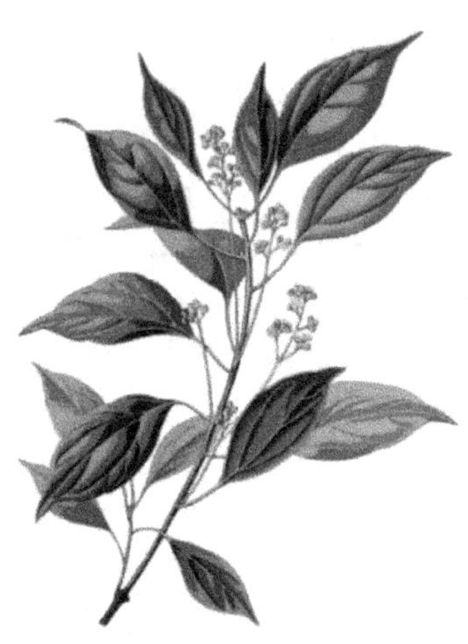

What's the Healthiest Diet to Follow?

There are so many diets out there and all sound promising. All make sense, but what is the best diet to stay healthy? What's the healthiest diet to follow? Is eating meat bad? Is it healthier to consume raw food? What about healthy carbs and fats? In this chapter, we will analyze all of these different diets and what's the most beneficial diet to follow.

Vegan Diet Plan:

A vegan diet excludes all animal products. Veganism is a way of living and is devoid of all animal products, including meat, eggs, and dairy. A vegan diet is based on foods such as vegetables, fruits, legumes, nuts, grains, and seeds. There are many benefits for vegans, and one of them is longevity. The second is happiness, as there is a plethora of studies that connect a good mood to vegetarianism. Next is weight loss, more energy, healthier skin, and so on...

So, what's Wrong with the Vegan Diet Plan?

Humans are closer to monkeys than cows. Vegetables are more difficult to digest raw and the reason is that humans do not have the cellulase enzyme. Animals that eat vegetables have this enzyme. So Humans do not manufacture the cellulase enzyme that helps to digest this type of fiber. So, while eating more vegetables is not a bad idea, eating mostly raw vegetables may be. A study found that a strict, raw vegan diet increased levels of homocysteine. High levels of homocysteine can damage the inside of your arteries.

Ketogenic Diet Plan:

A keto diet is a low carbs diet with moderate amounts of protein and healthy fats. The problem when you eat something high in carbs is that your body will produce glucose and insulin. When your body uses glucose as a primary energy, it is not burning fats. So, by lowering the intake of carbs, the body will use fats for fuel, and this state is known as ketosis. The ketones are produced from the breakdown of fats in the liver. The Keto diet it is used by many athletes and bodybuilders. There are many health benefits for people who follow the ketogenic plan diet. It reduces blood sugar and insulin levels, is good for weight loss, reduces blood pressure, and finally is a very effective treatment against metabolic syndrome.

So, what's Wrong with the Ketogenic Diet Plan?

Cells need oxygen and glucose, if we don't eat some healthy carbs, we can't be healthy. No carbs no longevity. Also, many nutritionists do not recommend the keto diet because it doesn't provide all the essential nutrients. Also, a diet high in meat and protein will be harmful to your health.

Paleo Diet Plan:

Paleo diet means giving up modern foods. So, the Paleo diet plan bans all forms of processed food, grains, dairy, and legumes, you must eat what a caveman ate and that's anything we could hunt or gather: Fish, meats, tubers, nuts, seeds, healthy fats, leafy greens, and veggies. Another thing about the Paleo diet is that you don't count calories you can eat until you're happy and full. Benefits: Cutting out processed foods improves health, protein builds muscles, you have fewer cravings, no calorie counting, more energy.

So, what's Wrong with the Paleo Diet Plan?

Paleo diet people declare that we shouldn't eat whole grains, dairy, and legumes, which in a way, is fine for people with celiac disease, lactose, and gluten sensitivity, but many studies have found that the benefits of grains and legumes outweigh their anti-nutrient content. Now about dairy, I will agree on some points, but not about healthy dairy products like feta or Greek yogurt. Also, as a big fan of the ancient Greek diet, I don't want to take those foods out of my diet. Another problem is also that the Paleo diet is mainly meat-based and a diet with too much animal fat, saturated fat, and protein is bad for your kidneys and impacts your cholesterol.

Raw Food Diet Plan:

A diet in that you eat almost everything unprocessed and uncooked. The raw food diet is also called raw foodism. With 70 percent fruits and 30 percent vegetables is a diet that obtains plenty of nutrients and your stomach digest system will thank you, as raw foods have more enzymes. This diet's concept is that humans were fruit-vegan animals closer to monkeys. So, this diet goes even farther from paleo. Without a doubt, the raw food diet has shown a lot of health benefits, and many people today use this diet as a cure for many diseases (including cancer) that modern medicine failed. This diet plan includes berries, fresh fruits, vegetables, sprouts, seeds, nuts, and herbs.

So, what's Wrong with the Raw Food Diet Plan?

It's challenging to stick to this diet. Even the biggest fans of this diet can't follow a 100-percent raw diet and most of them are only 75 to 80 percent raw-food eaters. That is because it's a hard diet and you miss a lot of flavors. Raw-food diet, in my opinion, is good for short-term fasting but not good for a long time. Another problem with this diet is muscle loss. Finally, even if the idea that monkeys are closer in nutrition to humans is correct, Humans have been eating cooked food for thousands of years, so I doubt that adapting raw food will be easy.

So, what's the Healthiest Diet to Follow?

Conclusion: So, if all of those diets have limitations and flaws, which is the healthiest diet to follow? For me, the best diet to follow is the diet that feet to your goals and style, but to be honest, I do a combination of all of them, and I created a super diet plan called: The wellness seeker diet. It's a combination of all the above plans.

The Wellness Seeker Diet:

The wellness seeker diet is all about balance. With the common sense and respect that Humans are omnivores for so many years, we need a modern balanced diet plan. It is a holistic diet that has to do with reality and modern life. Like mixed martial arts this diet is a combination of many diet plans. It is actually based on the Ancient Greek diet "Mediterranean diet", but with fasting breaks like days or weeks of fruit fasting or hours of intermittent fasting for cleansing and detoxing. Finally, even if the base is the Mediterranean diet, in the wellness seeker diet, we can eat food from many different world cuisines like Indian, Chinese, Japanese, French, and so on…

Wellness Seeker Diet General Rules:

Can I Consume Caffeine?

Caffeine in moderation it's ok, but only moderate, as daily caffeine consumption simply not working. Also, if you drink coffee every day, it's bad for your adrenal glands. Try to get caffeine only from healthy drinks like green tea, cocoa, or good-quality coffee. I consume caffeine three to four times a week, usually before training.

Can I Eat Carbs?

Carbohydrates are an essential part of a healthy diet, so yes, but only healthy carbs are allowed like: Fruits and berries, boiled potatoes, and sweet potatoes, whole grains include barley, black rice, oats, whole-wheat pasta, bread, legumes, etc. Try to eat clean, no processed foods, and no GMOs. It's better to eat carbs during the day and better as pre-workout and post-workout meals. Try also to avoid eating carbs together with protein and never eat fruits after or before your meal. You must consume fruits at least an hour after or before a meal.

Do we Count Calories?

If your goal is to lose weight and look better, then yes. Counting calories is very easy to do these days. There are so many useful apps and websites to help you with this.

What about Dairy?

Dairy is bad for our lymphatic system as it creates mucus, so it's better not to drink milk. If you like milk so much, then try to consume goat milk, which is closest to human milk. Now, because some dairy products have a lot of health benefits like probiotics, protein, healthy fats, etc. I recommend consuming dairy products in moderation. For cheese, I only recommend healthy choices like Organic, Feta, Pecorino Romano, Cottage Cheese, Ricotta, Aged Cheddar, Blue Cheese, Low-fat Swiss, Goat Cheese, etc. For yogurt, I only recommend Greek yogurt.

Can I Drink Alcohol?

Moderate alcohol consumption may have some substantial health benefits, so yes, alcohol under control will be ok for your diet. Enjoy a drink (Wine or Beer better) or two a day it's good for your well-being.

What about Protein?

Try to consume your proteins more from plant sources, if not, then second is fish and last is meat.

What about Cheat Meals?

Moderate and well-planned cheat meals (two times a week for example) will keep you healthy and teach your body to effectively manage extra food, so yes.

Eat Healthy Food at Ethnic Restaurants:

There are numerous healthy ethnic restaurants available. Eat some ethnic food, such as Indian, Chinese, or Japanese, since all of these kitchens have a lot of good ingredients like herbs, roots, and vegetables that we don't have in our kitchen.

Wellness Seeker Diet Combinations:

Eat Like a (Vegan):

Try to eat at least one meal of raw vegetables a day. Also, try to get your protein and amino acids from green vegetables instead of meat. We need less protein than most people think and an easy way to get this protein is from foods like nuts, cereals, vegetables, legumes, seeds, etc.

Eat More Raw Food:

As many experts believe, Humans are closer to Monkeys, and yes, many years ago we only ate fruits, seeds, and some raw vegetables. Raw food diet is one of the best diets to clean out toxins from the lymphatic system. That's why we need to fast at least two times a year for a week or more with 80 percent fruits and 20 percent greens. Also, if you eat for example four times a day, try two of your meals or snacks to be raw fruits or salads.

Try a Low Carb Diet:
The Keto diet is a low-carb diet. I don't recommend a full Keto diet and not all the time, as I like fruits and other healthy carbs to be a part of the wellness diet. Brain and muscles need carbs, so eating healthy carbs with your meals only before and after exercise or only in the morning is a very good strategy for losing weight.

Eat Like (Paleo):
Paleo is almost an omnivorous diet. So, from this diet, take only the good parts. Avoid all kinds of processed foods.

4 Simple Rules for those who Exercise:
Adopt the complete Wellness-Seeker diet when bulking up. Follow a low-carb Wellness-Seeker diet when maintaining. Follow a keto Wellness-Seeker diet when you are cutting. Utilize a raw food diet or fasting during cleansing.

Mediterranean Diet:

We all know that the Mediterranean diet has a lot of benefits, as this diet is renowned to be the healthiest diet in the world. When we talk about the Mediterranean diet, we mostly mean the diet in countries like Greece, Italy, France, and Spain. But all Mediterranean countries have influences and flavors from the Mediterranean diet. Countries like Slovenia, Croatia, Bosnia, Albania, Turkey, Syria, Lebanon, Israel, Tunisia, Egypt, Libya, Morocco, Algeria, Malta, and Cyprus share almost the same food ingredients and similar cuisine rules. The Mediterranean diet is my diet. The wellness seeker diet is based on a low-carb Mediterranean diet with short periods of intermittent fasting or water and dry fasting and some weeks of raw food diet for detoxification.

The Ancient Greek Diet and the Crete Diet:

In Ancient Greece, the diet was an important part of Greek philosophical thinking. A combination of pleasure and well-being. The main characteristic of the ancient Greek diet was simplicity. The meals of the day were mainly three and cereals were the basis of their diet. Most Greeks ate wheat and barley bread. A bread made from milk and barley flour was called MAZA and was eaten with cheese or honey. A great variety of vegetables was available in ancient Greece: Cabbage, onions, garlic, carrots, radishes, radishes, asparagus, and so on… Legumes like broad beans, lentils, peas, lupins, and chickpeas were also eaten daily. In ancient Greece, fruits were a significant part of the diet: Apples, pears, quinces, figs, pomegranate, grapes, apricots, melons, watermelons, cucumbers, lemons, oranges, and more. Greeks preferred fish more than meat and they knew how to cook seafood in many ways. Meat-eating was limited to public and private celebrations. Some experts say that the term "Mediterranean diet" refers to the diet of certain areas of the Mediterranean in the early 1960s, mainly Crete. Studies have shown that the expected life expectancy of the populations in these areas is one of the highest in the world, while coronary heart disease, certain types of cancer, and other chronic eating-related diseases were at very low levels. It is a fact that vegetables, fruits, whole grains, legumes, fish, healthy fats, and less red meat reduces Alzheimer's, heart disease, cancer, diabetes, and many other diseases.

Rules of the Mediterranean Diet:

Some general rules of the Mediterranean diet are: Avoid deli and processed meats, refined grains like white bread, and white pasta. Avoid bad refined oils, like vegetable canola, corn, and soybean oils. Finally, don't consume foods with added sugars like cakes, cookies, pastries, doughnuts, or sugar-sweetened drinks, such as processed fruit juices, energy drinks, soft drinks, and sports drinks. Eat in moderation seafood, eggs, and dairy. Try to limit those foods to two or three times per week. Eat red meat only rarely and red wine also in moderation. Eat more healthy fats, such as olive oil, nuts, and seeds, and also consume more fruits, vegetables, and whole grains. The Mediterranean benefits: It boosts brain power and reduces your risk of developing heart disease or cancer. It decreases your chances of developing chronic pain. The main point of this diet is to increase longevity.

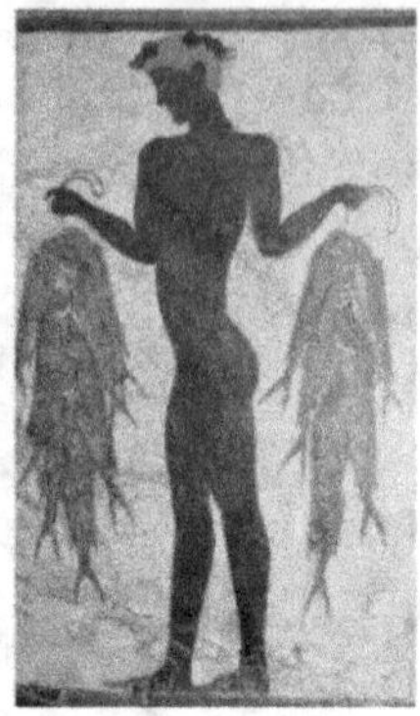

Greek Mountain Tea – Sideritis Scardica:

It is known as Sideritis Scardica, shepherd's tea, or Tsai Tou Vounou in Greek. This mountain tea is packed with flavonoids and antioxidants, and it is known as herbal medicine since ancient times. Hippocrates, Theophrastus, Dioscorides, and Galen describe it as a panacea. Studies have shown that it can prevent and even reverse Alzheimer's disease. Sideritis got its name from the Greek word Sidero **"iron"** because of the healing properties of the plant against wounds caused by iron weapons. These plants tend to live longer, more than two years. Sideritis Scardica grows in rocky places at high altitudes. The siderite genus plurality plant species (over 150 species), generally have small yellow flowers. Greece and Spain are the countries with the highest mountain tea consumption. It is often served, with honey and lemon. Traditionally in Greece, mountain tea is preferred for its beneficial effects on colds. It also helps with inflammation of the upper respiratory tract and anxiety. Is an immune system booster and helps with allergies and gastrointestinal disorders. Finally, Greek mountain tea is also famous for its miraculous properties against Alzheimer's disease. Research has found that mountain tea contains several components, mainly flavonoids, diterpenes, phenylpropane, iridoids, and monoterpenes. Of the approximately 17 species of Greece, only the six following are known: 1) Sideritis Athoa. 2) Sideritis Clandestina. 3) Sideritis Syriaca. 4) Sideritis Euboea. 5) Olympos Sideritis Scardica. 6) Parnassos Sideritis Raeseri.

Greek Sage:

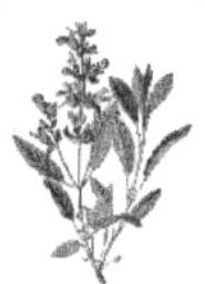

Known as Faskomilo in Greece. The extremely aromatic leaves of this plant are rich in antioxidants and used as a medicinal tea for sore throat, heartburn, insomnia, and hot flashes. It grows in Mediterranean countries like Greece, Spain, and Italy. It was considered a sacred herb by the ancient Greeks who dedicated it to Zeus. For the Latins was the plant of immortality. Greek Sage leaves are oblong, fluffy, and grey-green. In Greece, there are 20 different species of sage, and most of them are located in Southern Greece (Peloponnisos or the Islands). In the Latin language, "salvia" means "be healthy". Ancient Greek and Roman doctors like Dioscorides, Aetius, Hippocrates, and Galen, used Sage to heal snake bites and as a tonic for the mind and body. The Chinese call it Greek sprout, and in the Middle Ages, they exchanged three times the amount of the best quality tea with a little sage. Here are some benefits of Sage tea: It has anti-aging properties, improves memory, helps with liver debase, prevents diabetes, reduces anxiety, helps with skin problems, improves hair loss, reduces indigestion and dyspepsia, has anti-inflammatory properties, reduces sore throat, and has neurological benefits.

Mediterranean Honey:

The Mediterranean region has the best honey worldwide, an example is the Elvish honey. Research that is made on which Greek honey was highest in antioxidants levels has shown that oak honey was the number one, followed by fir honey, reiki honey, chestnut honey, pine honey, thyme honey, and orange honey.

Elvish Honey: I thought manuka honey was expensive until I found the Elvish honey which costs more than gold. Good honey is like good wine! Some like it strong, while others smooth and mild. Different countries produce different kinds of honey, but it all depends on the weather, the environmental conditions, and the bee species. But would you pay $6,800 just for honey? Some state that Elvish honey is the best honey in the world. Well, it is, without a doubt, the most expensive. Elvish honey comes from Turkey and is the most expensive honey in the world. This special honey is extracted from a 1,800-meter deep cave in Artvin city of the Saricayir valley. The prices are almost the same as those of white truffles! Elvish honey is produced in a natural way and without hives. The minerals from the cave naturally enhance the quality of the honey. Professional climbers help to extract Elvish Honey. It's amazing, that the first kilogram of this honey sold for 45,000 euros on the French stock exchange in 2009. The story starts in 2009, when a Turkish beekeeper named Gunduz, noticed some bees entering the cave of Saricayir valley. With the help of professional climbers, entered the cave and found 18 kilograms of honey plastered on its spherical walls. Later the honey was analyzed at a French lab and reported that it was seven years old and rich in minerals.

Reiki Honey: It is considered to be one of the best Mediterranean honeys! Because of the strong sweet-bitter flavor, it's not so famous. Reiki is completely different from all other kinds of honey that I know. It is also known as the Mediterranean Heather and it's made from three different plants: Erica carnea, Erica darleyensis, and Erica Manipuliflora. In the Greek language it is called: Ρεικόμελο (Reikomelo), and in Turkish: Püren Balı! The nutritional and therapeutic benefits of this honey are many. It is an immune system booster and is rich in iron and protein, can cure hay fever, helps with problems of the urinary system, and has antiseptic and diuretic properties. Finally, reiki honey has also the unique ability to lower cholesterol levels. Reiki most of the time crystallizes in one to three months. Erica is known as one of the best honeys in France.

Chios Mastic Gum:

The Mastiha of Chios is a natural antimicrobial agent and one of the best Mediterranean Superfoods. Mastic is a resin obtained from the mastic tree (Pistacia Lentiscus var. Chia). Originally it comes from the Greek island of Chios. Mastic has been used as chewing gum and a medicinal food in Mediterranean cultures for many centuries. Mastic appears as tear scratches and falls to the ground in drops. When the secretion of the Mastic tree has a sticky, clear liquid it is solidified into irregular shapes after 15-20 days. The form after solidification is crystalline and has a bitter taste. Chios Mastic can be used for stomach and intestinal ulcers, breathing problems, blood circulation, and bacterial infections. Chios gum might help reduce stomach acid and may protect the lining of the stomach and intestine. Mastic gum is also a natural Viagra for male sexuality. In the past, the Mastiha gum was administered to patients with renal insufficiency, and to patients with burns and skin diseases, as it has healing effects. Mastic antimicrobial action can eliminate H. pylori from the stomach in people who suffer from an infection caused by this bug. A study by scientists from the Hospital of Nottingham in Britain showed that even a small amount of Chios mastic (one gram per day) for two weeks can suppress the action of Helicobacter pylori and heal the ulcer.

Hippophae – Seabuckthorn Fruit:

Due to the fact that Hippophae is a genus of sea buckthorns, it is often referred to as sea buckthorn. Hippophae was consumed by the army of Great Alexander. Hippo in ancient Greece means horse and phae means bright, so Hippo-phae means bright horse. Alexander noticed that sick horses that ate Sea Buckthorn were recovering faster and had more power. According to studies Hippophae has anticancer properties, as it is rich in vitamin C content, can boost the immune system, can reduce LDL cholesterol levels, is good for the skin, and can help with weight loss.

Feta Cheese:

According to many studies is the world's healthiest cheese and is a must if you follow the Mediterranean diet plan. The original Greek feta it's made with goat or sheep's milk and not cow's milk. As it is made from unpasteurized milk, feta is packed with Probiotics and is high in protein content, phosphorous, calcium, vitamin B12, and riboflavin. It lowers the risk of Type 2 Diabetes, is good for bone health, it fights anemia, and it's beneficial for building muscles.

Olives and Olive Oil:

Olives are in our life for more than 7,000 years and are an essential part of the Mediterranean diet. It is an antioxidant-rich food with antimicrobial properties that protect against cancer, reduce blood pressure, protect against ulcers, improve memory, and may help prevent strokes. Extra virgin olive oil is rich in healthy monounsaturated fats and has strong anti-inflammatory and antibacterial properties.

Capers:

Another Mediterranean Superfood, capers are high in polyphenols and antioxidants. With so many antimicrobial properties, capers can cure infections. In ancient Greece, caper was used as bloating and flatulence remedy. Today studies have shown that Caper is good for diabetes and weight loss, is protecting from allergies, boosts immunity, and helps with bad cholesterol LDL.

Rosemary:

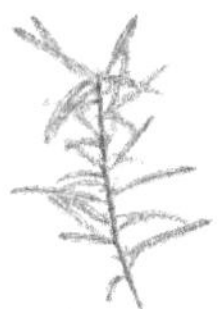

Rosemary is a herb native to the Mediterranean region, it has antioxidant, antimicrobial, anti-inflammatory, and antispasmodic properties. Ancient Greeks used the plant for assisting memory and stimulating the brain. Research has shown that Rosemary can protect liver cells, lower blood sugar, may improve mood and memory, protects vision, and promotes digestion.

<h2 style="text-align:center">Oregano:</h2>

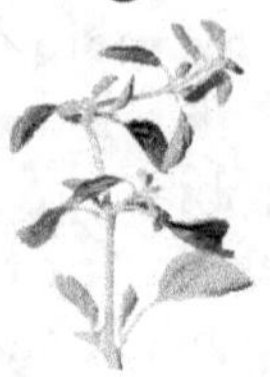

Oregano is packed with antioxidants. The oregano essential oil is one of the best Mother nature's antibiotics and has anti-viral, anti-inflammatory, anti-bacterial, and anti-fungal properties. It may help lower cholesterol, could help with pain, has cancer-fighting properties, boosts immunity, and aids in digestion.

<h2 style="text-align:center">Thyme:</h2>

Thyme is another herbal medicine from the mint family. Like oregano, thyme is a natural antibiotic and has anti-inflammatory, anti-bacterial, and anti-fungal properties. It helps fight sore throats, can help with intestinal infections, can boost immunity, and finally, can help to reduce blood pressure and cholesterol levels.

<h2 style="text-align:center">Parsley:</h2>

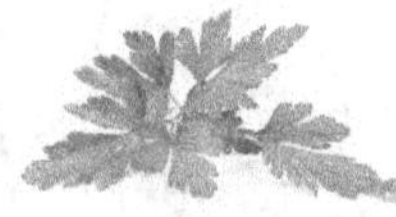

Another super-food native to the Mediterranean region. Is highly nutritious and has many healing properties. Is a rich source of antioxidants like volatile oils and flavonoids. This plant prevents cancer and rheumatoid arthritis. Promotes kidney cleanses, protects against diabetes, improves bone health, and relieves flatulence.

Linden:

Tilia is famous for its medicinal effects. Linden tea has a high concentration of phytonutrients, flavonoids, and powerful antioxidants like Tiliroside and kaempferol. Tilia Cordata or Tilia Platyphyllos is known for its soothing and relaxing abilities. It is the best beverage to drink late in the evening as it helps the body to relax from tension. Linden is a beautiful tree, reaching 30 m high and living up to 200 years. Tilia tea has a lot of ways to promote health, is anti-hypertensive, diuretic, and reduces colds & fevers. The name "Tilia" is Latin and derived from the ancient Greek word "Ptelea". The high concentration of flavonoids and phytonutrients is what makes this tea so special! The leaves of the linden tree are heart-shaped and the flowers are white-yellow and have a very sweet fragrance. It thrives in areas with a temperate climate and mountainous terrain. Tilia flowers are the most commonly used part of these trees. The northern Europeans used the inner bark of the tree to create ropes, shoes, fishing nets, and other objects. Linden flower honey is very good for your health and you can find good quality Linden flower honey mainly in northern Greece. In Greek mythology, Linden was the mother of the centaur Chiron. Chiron was a famous Centaur, healer, and educator. Other Linden flower tea benefits: Tilia reduces high blood pressure, promotes rest, strengthens the immune system, relieves anxiety, detoxifies the body, prevents cancer, and is beneficial to the heart, lungs, digestion, and kidney stones.

Stinging Nettle:

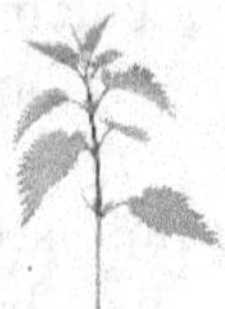

Nettle tea was used in ancient Greece and Rome for the treatment of a variety of health conditions. This super herb contains many nutrients like vitamins, minerals, amino acids, healthy fats, polyphenols, and pigments. Today is mostly used to flush away toxins, soothe allergies, for the treatment of sore stiff joints and muscles, and prostate health.

Bay Leaf:

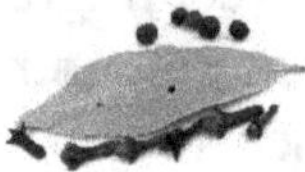

Native to the Mediterranean, this herb has been around for centuries. This leaf is used in Greek and Italian cooking for its distinctive flavor and fragrance. Bay leaf has antimicrobial and antioxidant qualities and can be useful for diabetics. It may help to fight cancer, aid digestion, and may prevent candida.

Digestive Enzymes:

As I'm also suffering from time to time with GERD and gastritis, I have found natural ways to control these symptoms. Nutrition, exercise, and supplements like probiotics are some of them. But one of the best secrets for all these diseases is the digestive enzymes. Most people who suffer from acid reflux believe that the problem is excessive acid, but in some cases, the problem is low stomach acid (hypochlorhydria). One of the best ways to produce enzymes in your body is by eating raw food, like fruits and vegetables. As we grow older food becomes harder to absorb. Enzymes help us to break down nutrients easily. Probiotics and digestive enzymes at the same time can work as a medicine for many diseases like IBS, Gastritis, GERD, and so on... These supplements can treat symptoms like gas, belching, bloating, constipation, diarrhea, and heartburn.

Top Digestive Enzymes:

Amylase converts carbohydrates and starches into sugars for energy.

Lipase converts fat and triglycerides into essential fatty acids.

Protease breakdown proteins into smaller polypeptides or single amino acids.

Lactase converts lactose into simpler sugar forms like glucose and galactose.

Nucleases are produced by the pancreas and break down bonds between nucleic acids.

Bromelain is an enzyme found in pineapple used for reducing inflammation.

Pepsin also breaks down proteins into smaller peptides. **Papain** extracted from the papaya and helps to break proteins down into smaller protein fragments.

The supplementation of digestive enzymes is not a bad idea, but in my opinion, it is preferable not to depend on them. When we take probiotics and enzymes from supplements, we simply make our bodies lazy to produce by themselves. Instant of probiotics, eat prebiotic foods like bananas and asparagus and for digestive enzymes, eat more raw food. Now, for people that have problems with milk, coffee, or any other trigger, just try to avoid these foods and give your body some time to heal. I take probiotics and digestive enzymes only if I have Gastritis and GERD attacks. Here are some foods that contain digestive enzymes: Pineapples, papayas, bananas, mangoes, avocados, ginger, kefir, kimchi, miso, kiwifruit, and sauerkraut.

Top Super Fruits and Super Berries:

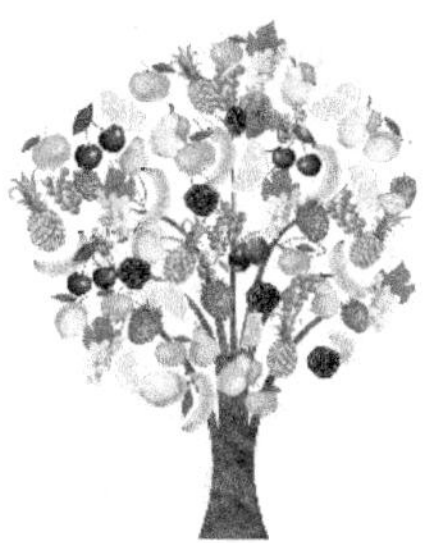

We all need fruits in our diet, as they are low in calories, and high in fiber. For sure, fruits are the best source of vitamins, minerals, and antioxidants. We've all heard about superfoods lately, so here are some superfruits and super-berries for you. Most of the fruits are healthy but only some come with these "superpowers".

Maqui Berry:

This super berry is a rich source of antioxidants (anthocyanins). It grows primarily in Andean Patagonia, between the Chilean and Argentinian Mountains. The Mapuche Indians used Maqui for strength and stamina and to treat fever, ulcers, diarrhea, and hemorrhoids. Consuming maqui berries or their juice boosts metabolism, has anti-aging properties and can treat diabetics, cardiovascular problems, and kidney problems.

Acai Berry:

Acai berries come from the acai palm trees that are native to the rainforests of South America. This berry is often used by alternative medical practitioners for many different health benefits. It boosts energy, promotes heart health, helps with weight loss, high cholesterol, and erectile dysfunction, is good for the skin, it stops bad cell proliferation, improves mental function, and is good for detoxification.

Cherimoya - Custard Apple:

Custard Apple: Note: The seeds of Cherimoya are quite toxic (cyanide), I was accidentally eating them and I was ill for two days. Custard apples are native to South America, are rich in antioxidants and have anti-cancer properties, can improve vision, treat diabetes, boosts immunity, and prevent arthritis.

Soursop – Graviola Fruit:

Soursop is a superfruit with plenty of vitamin C and many health benefits. Graviola belongs to the same family as Custard Apple and is native to the Caribbean, Central, and South America. Soursop has similar health benefits to Cherimoya fruit and has many anti-cancer properties.

Camu Camu Berry:

Another vitamin C Super-Berry. Camu berry comes from the Amazonian rainforest of Peru. One teaspoon of Camu Camu could provide 685 mg of vitamin C. Did you knew that according to a study taking 500–1,000 mg of vitamin C increased glutathione levels in white blood cells in healthy adults? Camu Camu berry prevents aging, boosts the immune system, protects against cancer, helps with weight loss and muscle growth.

Durian:

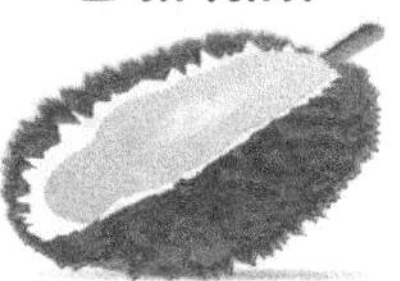

Native to southeast Asia is one of the best fruits for depression. Some chemicals in this fruit like the amino acid tryptophan are converted to serotonin. Durian will give you hotness, and has some aphrodisiac effects. Southeast Asians referred to Durian as the "King of Fruits." It is a good source of energy, promotes bone health, helps with insomnia, and reduces blood pressure.

Noni:

It is also known as Indian mulberry and is native to Indonesia and Australia. Noni juice is famous for its medicinal properties and studies showed that it can be a wonder for your health. Noni has anti-aging properties, it prevents cancer, may boost immunity, may kill bacteria, fungi, and parasites, can treat fever, protects heart health, and may lower cholesterol.

Hippophae:

As it is mentioned above, according to studies Hippophae has anticancer properties, as it is rich in vitamin C content, can boost the immune system, can reduce LDL cholesterol levels, is a skin healer, and can help with weight loss.

Amla:

I saw Amla berries for the first time in Nepal. Amla is called Indian Gooseberry as it is native to India. Amla was used for more than 5,000 years in Ayurvedic medicine. These berries are packed with whole food vitamin C and bioflavonoids. Amla helps in boosting the immune system, acts as a diuretic, increases protein synthesis, reduces bad cholesterol, has Anti-ageing properties, and finally, is good for weight loss.

Red Grapes:

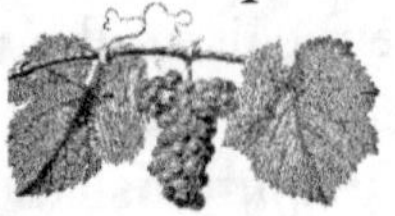

One more superfruit, for me, Red Grapes are the best fruits for detoxification, especially if you mix them with a raw food diet. Women on the Greek island of Crete spend weeks eating only red grapes to detoxify their lymphatic system. Grapes have a lot of health benefits. The skin and seeds of the red grapes contain resveratrol, a strong antioxidant with anti-aging, antibacterial, and antiviral properties.

Red Jujube Dates:

This super fruit is also called Chinese red date, as it's native to China. It's been used in Traditional Chinese Medicine for more than 3,000 years and it contains half the calories and sugar of the regular date. This fruit helps with insomnia and promotes high-quality sleep, regulates circulation, boosts immunity, improves digestion, and prevents cancer.

Tamarind:

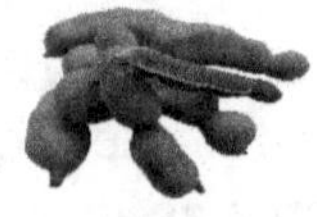

It is a delicious sweet-sour fruit. It is originally from Africa but can be found in many tropical regions. In Southeast Asia, it is used in cooking. This tropical superfruit has a lot of medicinal properties. Improves circulation, is good for weight loss, has anti-fungal and antibacterial effects, can reduce LDL cholesterol, is good for the digestive system, and has anti-aging properties.

Cape Gooseberries:

I do a lot of superfood smoothies with Cape Gooseberries when I need a high dose of vitamin C. Also known as Inca berry, golden berries, and Rasbhari in India. Cape Gooseberries are packed with nutrients and have antimicrobial, anticancer, antipyretic, and anti-inflammatory properties.

Schisandra Berries:

Native to China and Russia, Schisandra is an adaptogenic herb used in traditional Chinese medicine for many years now. They are also called the Five Flavor Berry, as it tastes sweet, sour, bitter, salty, and even spicy. These berries reduce inflammation, boost energy, improve liver function, protect the skin, protect vision, improve mental performance, and increase libido.

Longan Fruit:

It's also called euphoria fruit as it has some anti-depression effects. Longan fruit is native to Southeast Asia. I ate a lot of them in Thailand. Longan fruit belongs to the family of soapberries (lychee, salt lime, ackee, and guarana). It's been used for many years in traditional medicine as it contains anti-aging properties, has anticancer effects, reduces stress, and improves memory.

Chokeberry Aronia:

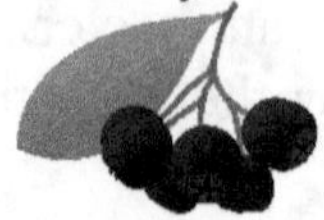

Chokeberries are native to North America and have three times more antioxidants and phytonutrients than blueberries. It is one of the most potent super-berries because it has anti-cancer properties, anti-diabetic effects, boosts immunity, aids in weight loss, and regulates blood pressure.

Acerola Cherries:

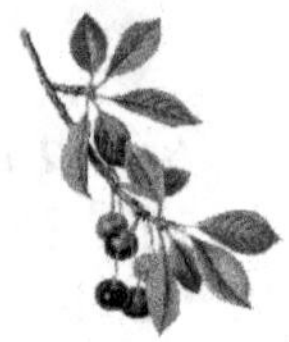

This superfruit is native to South and Central America. Since a single Acerola cherry can usually contain more than 1000 mg of vitamin C, most people use it to treat the common cold. It prevents diabetes and liver damage, improves cardiovascular health, promotes strong bones, and prevents aging.

Elderberry:

This dark purple super berry is one of the most used medicinal plants in the world. Elderberry teas and syrups are the best remedies in cold and flu season, Elderberry is high in antioxidants, is good for heart health, supports the immune system, is a diuretic, is good for allergies, and promotes mental health.

Blackcurrant:

This super berry is native to parts of Europe and Asia. Black currant has a lot of good vitamins, essential minerals, and antioxidants. It keeps our cardiovascular system healthy, can help fight infections, helps in controlling high blood pressure, is great for hair and skin, may help with insomnia, and improves the digestive system.

Baobab Fruit:

The baobab is known as the "Tree of Life" and comes from Africa, but it is also native to Arabia, and Australia. Inside baobab fruits, you will find only a dry powder, that contains important minerals and vitamins. Baobab fruit prevents arthritis, builds bone strength, boosts the immune system, supports heart health, prevents cancer, and lowers inflammation.

Lucuma:

Native to Peru, this fruit used for a long time now as a low GI sweetener. The "gold of the Incas" contains a lot of antioxidants, minerals, and vitamins that may benefit blood sugar control, supports the immune system, improves the skin, reduces inflammation, and promote heart health.

Goji Berries:

Native to Asia, particularly China, it is also known as wolfberries. Goji berry is famous as a medicinal herb for more than 2,000 years. These berries provide high levels of antioxidants, protect against age-related eye diseases, increases testosterone, fight cancer, promote healthy skin, support the immune system, and prevent liver damage.

Avocado:

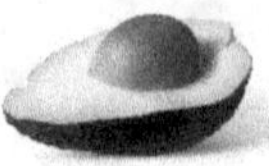

It is considered one of the world's healthiest superfoods. Avocado is native to Mexico and Central America. Its nutrient-rich, it's good for the heart, eyes, and liver, contains anti-aging and anti-cancer properties, and is good for depression, and digestion.

Mangosteen:

Native to Southeast Asia, Mangosteen is rich in antioxidants, vitamins, and xanthones. I saw this exotic superfruit for the first time in Thailand. Mangosteen has anti-cancer and anti-bacterial effects. Can boosts immunity, regulates blood pressure, helps with diabetes and skin care, protects the heart, and helps with weight loss.

Blueberries:

We all know Blueberries as a superfruit. This berry is high in antioxidants and flavonoids like anthocyanin. Blueberries improve lung function, are good for managing diabetes, they are lowering blood pressure, are good for the bones, they protecting against heart disease, and can help with muscle recovery.

Pomegranate:

This sweet-sour fruit has some amazing medicinal powers. Studies have shown that Pomegranate has a lot of health benefits for our body. Pomegranate has antibacterial and antiviral properties.

The seeds of this fruit can protect our body from cancerous cells. Pomegranate juice can lower the blockage in the arteries and helps with osteoarthritis and blood pressure. Finally, can treat anemia, and erectile dysfunction.

Grapefruit and Pomelo:

Pomelo is a tropical cousin of the grapefruit and they both belong to the giant citrus family. Actually, it's the largest of all citrus fruits and that's why the scientific name is Citrus maxima. Like most citrus fruits, grapefruits and pomelos are high in vitamin C. Pomelos originated in Southeast Asia. I tried for the first-time pomelo in Laos, "called Somo in Lao". Due to their high bioflavonoid content, citrus fruits protect against uti and are beneficial for the heart, anemia, and allergies. can aid in shedding pounds, strengthen hair, and eventually, protect against the flu, colds, and osteoporosis.

Best Probiotic and Prebiotic Foods:

If your goal is to have good stomach and gut health then you need both, Prebiotics and Probiotics. Now, to the question of what you need more, prebiotics or probiotics, I must answer that prebiotics are for sure more important. Prebiotics are actually served as food for probiotics. Prebiotics will help our body to produce more probiotics. Eating prebiotics will help probiotics multiply and remain in our intestines. Probiotics, on the other hand, are live good bacteria that keep balance in our digestive system and occur in many fermented foods. There are many types of probiotics like Bifidobacterium, Lactobacillus, and Saccharomyces Boulardii yeast-type bacteria. Different probiotics have different effects.

Top Prebiotic Foods:

Legumes: Lentils, black beans, kidney beans, peas, soybeans, and chickpeas are rich in prebiotic carbohydrates.

Oats: Yes, whole oats are a good source of prebiotic fiber. This prebiotic grain has a lot of health benefits.

Bananas: Another great source of prebiotic fiber is bananas. Studies have shown that bananas reduce bloating and increase healthy gut bacteria.

Berries: Blueberries, blackberries, raspberries, grapes, goji berries, bilberries, strawberries, and acai berries are all-powerful prebiotic foods.

Artichokes: The delicious artichokes are an excellent source of nutrients, rich in antioxidants and prebiotic carbohydrates.

Asparagus: Raw asparagus is packed with good vitamins, and minerals, and is another great source of prebiotics.

Dandelion Greens: Dandelion greens are delicious and also a good source of prebiotic fiber called inulin, a group of naturally occurring polysaccharides.

Garlic: Raw garlic is a great source of copper, manganese, selenium, vitamin B6, vitamin C, and prebiotic fiber.

Onions: Onions are another high prebiotic food. Eating onions provide a lot of nutrients and have many possible health benefits.

Leeks: Like garlic and onion, leeks are a member of the allium family and also one of the best sources of prebiotics.

Apple Cider Vinegar: Many people say that Apple cider vinegar is a probiotic. No, apple cider vinegar is not a probiotic, but it is full of prebiotics and contains pectin, which feeds probiotics in the gut.

Top Probiotic Foods:

Yogurt: Yogurt especially Lassi or Greek Yogurt is packed with beneficial probiotics. The probiotics in yogurt are Lactobacillus Bulgaricus and Streptococcus Thermophilus.

Kimchi: Kimchi is packed with delicious spicy flavor, beneficial nutrients, and is one of the oldest Korean vegetable fermented foods.

Pickles: Note that pickles made with vinegar do not contain any live probiotics. Fermented pickles, on the other hand, are packed with good bacteria for your gut.

Natto: Natto is considered a superfood and is very nutritious. This Japanese fermented soybean healthy food has some bacteria called Bacillus subtilis that help to synthesize enzymes. These enzymes have a lot of benefits for our health.

Sauerkraut: Sauerkraut is a famous fermented cabbage and one of the healthiest probiotic-rich foods. It contains far more lactobacillus than yogurt, which improves the balance of good bacteria in your gut.

Kombucha: Kombucha is a popular fermented tea and another rich source of probiotics. Some said that have originated in China during the Tsin dynasty.

Miso: I think most of you have already tried the delicious fermented Japanese miso soup. Miso has both prebiotic and probiotic qualities.

Traditional Buttermilk: Buttermilk is a fermented drink and a good source of probiotics. Living lactic acid bacteria gives traditional buttermilk its sour taste.

Some Types of Cheese: Feta, gouda, mozzarella, cheddar, cottage cheese, and blue cheese are full of probiotics and some other beneficial bacteria that offer many health benefits.

Kefir: kefir or kephir is fermented milk and is actually a better source of probiotics than yogurt or kombucha. Kephir contains up to 60 strains of bacteria and yeasts.

Best Super Seeds for your Health:

According to some philosophers, seeds represent life. That's why we have to find the best seeds for our health. Seeds are a great snack to fight hunger with a lot of benefits. These top super seeds are rich in minerals, proteins, vitamins, enzymes, and fatty acids. So, in a way, are a must-have on our nutrition plan. I recommend eating seeds raw to get all the nutrition benefits. If you soak the seeds is even better, as toxic substances can be eliminated and can be easily digested.

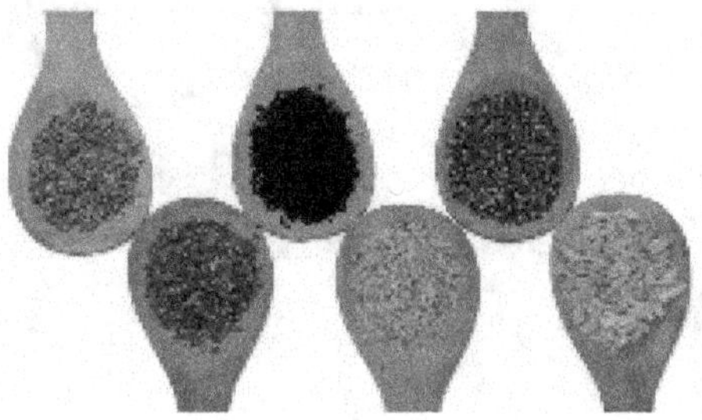

Top Super Seeds and their Benefits:

Cannabis Seeds:

Cannabis seeds are a superfood that is high in protein and a good source of omega-3 fatty acids. Cannabis seeds contain all 20 amino acids. Protein, helps in building muscles, so sprinkling cannabis seeds on your food or in your beverage after exercise helps your muscles to stimulate. Nutritional value: 90 calories per 2 tablespoons, 6 grams of fat, 2 grams of fiber, 5 grams of protein, and 4 grams of carbs.

Pumpkin seeds:

Pumpkin seeds are the best seeds for your health. We all know lentils and spinach as sources of iron, but pumpkin seeds are very rich in iron too. These seeds are also rich in magnesium another important metal that helps our body to produce energy. Nutritional value: 158 calories per 2 tablespoons, 14 grams of fat, 2 grams of fiber, 9 grams of protein, and 0 grams of carbs.

Sesame Seeds:

Sesame Seeds contain linolenic acid, which is part of the omega-6 fatty acids that can help to regulate cholesterol. So yes, sesame is very good for your heart. If you strain the seeds, you make Greek tahini, an immune-boosting heart protector. Nutritional value: 103 calories per 2 tablespoons, 9 grams of fat, 2 grams of fiber, 3 grams of protein, and 6 grams of carbs.

Chia Seeds:

Chia seeds are one of the best super-seeds out there. They can stick to your teeth if you consume them in dry form so it is always better if you soak them. If you consume chia often, you will soon notice the health benefits such as an increase in your energy levels and an improvement in the digestive process. Nutritional value: 138 calories per 2 tablespoons, 9 grams of fat, 10 grams of fiber, 5 grams of protein, and 2 grams of carbs.

Flax Seeds:

Rich in omega-3 fatty acids and iron. Flax seeds are really good for the heart and can reduce inflammation that leads to various diseases. Flaxseeds have a strong flavor and can transform into a form of smooth gel when mixed with some liquid. Thirty grams of flaxseeds contain about 12 grams of fatty acids, and about 1/4 of the recommended daily magnesium intake. Nutritional value: 110 calories per 2 tablespoons, 9 grams of fat, 6 grams of fiber, 4 grams of protein, and 4 grams of carbs.

Sunflower Seeds:

Sunflower seeds are also among the healthiest seeds. About half a cup of sunflower seeds contains more than 100% of the daily recommended dose of vitamin E. The seeds also contain alpha-tocopherol, a powerful antioxidant that protects the body's cells from ultraviolet radiation damage. It is also an important source of an amino acid called phenylalanine, which is used by the brain as an antidepressant and keeps us alert. Sunflower seeds can be used in many ways. They can be eaten raw or baked, added to salads, bread, and so on... Nutritional value: 62 calories per 2 tablespoons, 5 grams of fat, 1 gram of fiber, 2 grams of protein, and 4 grams of carbs.

Quinoa Seeds:

There are 3 types of quinoa seeds that we can find today, red, white, and black. Quinoa comes from South America (Peru, Chile, Bolivia). For thousands of years, it was the basic diet of the Incas. It has twice the protein content compared to rice and is richer in minerals such as calcium, magnesium, and manganese.

Finally, Quinoa has a good level of B complex vitamins, vitamin E, and iron. Nutritional value: 80 calories per 2 tablespoons, 2 grams of fat, 2 grams of fiber, 2 grams of protein, and 14 grams of carbs.

Pine Seeds:

We usually consume pine seeds after they fall from the tree and open from the sun. We can eat them raw or baked. Ancient Greeks and Romans appreciated their rich nutritional value and they considered as a symbol of fertility. Pine seeds are rich in vitamins B1 and E, copper, iron, omega-3 fatty acids, magnesium, manganese, and zinc. Nutritional value: 130 calories per 2 tablespoons, 14 grams of fat, 0 grams of fiber, 3 grams of protein, and 3 grams of carbs.

Watermelon Seeds:

Watermelon seeds are also at the top of this list. Rich in Vitamin C, Pantothenic Acid, Biotin, Vitamin A (Carotenoids), Vitamin B1, Vitamin B6, fatty acids and essential proteins, magnesium, manganese, iron, potassium, copper, zinc, phosphorus, thiamine, niacin, and folic acid. Nutritional value: 76 calories per 2 tablespoons, 6 grams of fat, 0 grams of fiber, 4 grams of protein, and 2 grams of carbs.

Top Healthiest Legumes:

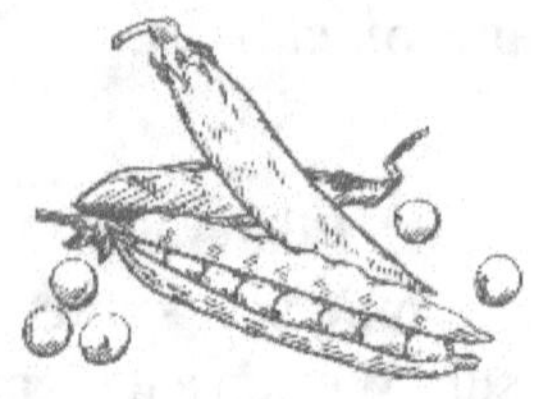

Legumes are high in protein and are heart-healthy vegetable plants. Legumes are a great replacement for meat as a source of protein. Are high in fiber, antioxidants, and minerals without the saturated fat found in most animal proteins.

Lentils:

Lentils are one of the World's healthiest foods and can help with many serious medical problems. The benefits of lentils are well known in Asian countries like India and Nepal, and in Mediterranean countries like Greece, Italy, Libano, etc. I consume lentils from a very young age, as lentils are a very common food in the Mediterranean. Lentils are quick and easy to prepare and don't take so much time to cook compared to other types of beans.

Nutrition Facts of Lentils:

Lentils are first on my top healthiest legumes list. Rich in fiber, with lean protein, phosphorus, manganese, iron, potassium, folate, calcium, zinc, Vitamin D, K, C, B6, and niacin.

One cup of Lentils Contains About:
36 percent of phosphorus.
37 percent of iron.
21 percent of potassium.
49 percent of manganese.
90 percent of folate.
18 percent of vitamin B6.
22 percent of thiamin.
63 percent of Fiber.

Lentils Benefits:

Heart and Cholesterol: Lentils help to reduce blood cholesterol. Research at the American Heart Association showed that increased fiber intake can reduce LDL ("bad") cholesterol levels.

Cancer: Lentils have a great potential to control cancer growth.
Research studies have shown that Selenium (a mineral found in lentils) decreases tumor growth.

Controls Diabetes: Soluble fiber helps stabilize blood sugar levels. A study showed that dietary fiber helps in controlling blood sugar levels.

Increases Energy: Lentils can increase your energy, as it is a good source of fiber, complex carbohydrates, and iron, which transport oxygen throughout your body.

Weight Loss: Lentils are low in calories and regular consumption of lentils can help in weight control and increase satiety.

Peas:

Peas are my favorite source of high-quality plant protein. I love a Greek food recipe that's made with peas, artichokes, and dill. Often regarded as a superfood, peas are a good source of dietary fiber, Vitamin K, Vitamin A, iron, thiamin, folate, Vitamin C, and manganese. Green peas have many health benefits. Better digestion, good for weight loss, increases bone strength, regulates blood sugar, lower bad cholesterol, fights inflammation, improves immunity, and oxygen levels in the blood.

Peanuts:

Peanuts originated in South America. Eating these legumes is associated with many health benefits, especially for the heart as they are packed with heart-healthy monounsaturated fats, minerals, antioxidants, and vitamins. Peanuts may lower bad cholesterol (LDL), aid in weight loss, lower blood sugar levels, reduce the risk of Alzheimer's disease, protect against gallstones, and, finally, reduce cancer risk.

Beans:

Beans are the seeds of flowering plants in the Fabaceae family. They are over 400 different types of edible beans grown throughout the world and they for sure are among the top healthiest legumes. Some famous beans are Black-Eyed Beans, Red Beans, Kidney Beans, Black Beans, Soybeans, Garbanzo Beans, Pinto Beans, Navy Beans, Fava Beans, Cannellini Beans, and Lima Beans. As beans are high in sulfur like all the other legumes, must be soaked overnight prior to cooking. Beans are rich in complex carbs and are also an excellent source of fiber, protein, B vitamins, potassium, folate, iron, potassium, selenium, vitamin K, calcium, thiamine, magnesium, manganese, zinc, and copper. Beans provide myriad health benefits. A study has shown that eating beans four times per week reduced heart disease risk by 22 percent. Beans can reduce LDL ("bad") cholesterol and blood sugar levels, are good for weight loss, prevent fatty liver, and more. I can't write about all the beans available, so I'll stick to my personal favorite.

Chickpeas:

Chickpeas are also known as garbanzo beans. These beans are very famous in the Mediterranean, middle east, and Indian cuisine. Commonly chickpeas are white-beige, but there are other varieties like black, red, and green.

Chickpeas Benefits:

Diabetes: According to a study, chickpeas serve as a diabetic superfood.

Digestive Tract Support: The fiber in Chickpeas can actually support digestive tract function.

Bone Health: Chickpeas are perfect for bone structure and strength.

Good for Heart: Chickpeas lower blood pressure and are very good for the heart! Foods with high-fiber like chickpeas help to prevent heart disease.

Antioxidants: Chickpeas are famous in terms of their antioxidant composition.

Anti-Cancer Effects: Garbanzo beans might also offer protection against certain types of cancer.

Cholesterol: Chickpeas can help to lower your (LDL) cholesterol in the blood.

The Best Mushrooms for your Health:

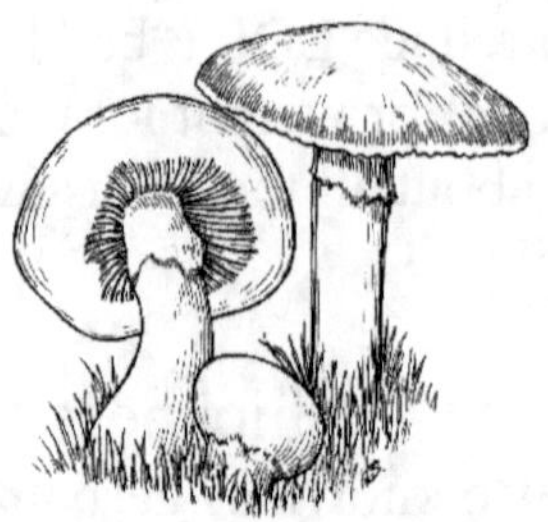

I have been always fascinated by Mushrooms. Mushrooms are packed with nutrients and are rich in fiber, protein, vitamins, minerals, and antioxidants. They were used as food, medicine, and spiritual booster for centuries. From puffballs to truffles, there are so many different kinds of mushrooms for different uses. We have delicious fungi like cremini and portobellos and more medicinal like cordyceps, reishi, chaga, and shiitake. Of course, there are also the psychedelic-magic mushrooms that are still a mystery in many ways. Mushroom DNA is more similar to mammals than plants and for that reason, fungi activate all the healthy adaptogenic properties of the human body. Mushrooms were used in many ancient cultures. The psychedelic effect of mushrooms for example was well known in ancient Greece and Egypt, but also in Mayan and Aztec civilizations. Mushrooms are edible fungi but remember all mushrooms are fungi, but not all fungi are mushrooms. Here are the healthiest mushrooms to add to your diet and used as a superfood.

Shiitake Mushrooms:

Shiitake mushrooms are one of the best foods to add to your diet! These mushrooms contain some chemical compounds that protect your DNA from oxidative damage. Today modern science has proved that the Shiitake mushroom support immune function, promotes heart health, reduces the risk of prostate cancer, helps prevent gingivitis, and boosts energy and brain function.

Shitake Mouthwash:

A lot of people are saying an apple a day keeps the doctor away, but what about a Mushroom a day keeps the dentist away? Today modern science is here to prove the amazing properties of Shiitake mushroom as a mouthwash, against plaque, gingivitis, and Gum Disease. Chinese medicine used shiitake mushrooms for centuries to treat many different diseases. Shiitake mushrooms are a very popular food source in Asia and are the third most widely distributed mushroom in the world. These mushrooms are for sure a superfood as they contain many chemical compounds that protect your DNA from oxidative damage.

The Evidence:

The first time I saw the dental benefits of Shiitake mushrooms was in the Superfood series. University College London is one of the many UK Universities that study Shiitake. According to the research of Dr. Spate, Shiitake mouthwash increased the population of good bacteria in the teeth and at the same time lowered the numbers of pathogenic organisms. Here is another study, researchers from the Italy's University of Verona did the same study and found that Shiitake Mushroom extracts appear to kill oral bad bacteria.

The problem with our common strong mouthwashes is that can kill most bacteria, which means they can also throw off the balance of good bacteria. Kate from the Superfood series made the experiment herself and found the same results.

The Experiment:

I did the same experiment two weeks ago, as I had really bad pain in my gums. That was the perfect time to see if the Shiitake mouthwash works. For seven days, I washed my teeth twice a day with Shiitake. The pain was less severe for the first three days, but by the fourth day, I was feeling much better. For sure, the Shiitake-mouthwash helps a lot with gum disease.

Shiitake Mouthwash Recipe:

All you need is a Blender, some water, and some Shiitake mushrooms. Mix them for about 10 seconds until the mushrooms melted. That's it. Your Shiitake mouthwash against plaque, gingivitis, and gum disease is ready. I have to warn you that it has a terrible taste, so be prepared.

Shiitake Mushrooms for Libido:

As I said, I tried recently a mouthwash recipe with shiitake mushrooms, and during my experiment, I noticed that my sex drive also increased. After this, I made some research and I found that mushrooms in general, and mainly Shiitake used as a powerful sexual stimulating tonic. Asian tradition recommends the use of shiitake for high blood pressure, heart disease, obesity, and sexual dysfunction. I put Shiitake Mushrooms in my diet for a week and the results were amazing! Mushrooms can improve your sex life magically. Shiitake is known as a vasodilator; it reduces the blocking of arteries and increases the blood flow of the penis. The zinc in shiitake mushrooms promotes immune function, but Zinc is also tagged as the ultimate sex mineral. Zinc-rich mushrooms are found to improve sperm count and fertility in males. So, cure your erectile dysfunction naturally with Mushrooms.

Reishi or Lingzhi Mushrooms:

Lingzhi mushroom is a woody fungus with a bitter taste. It is called Reishi in Japanese and Ling Zhi in the Chinese language, but most people know it as Ganoderma Lucidum (Greek-Latin)! Reishi mushroom might be the most dynamic superfood for longevity ever. In China Lingzhi is one of the oldest symbols of well-being and longevity. Was first mentioned in Cao Zhi's poem, as lingcao "magic herb". This Mushroom is used by Taoists and Buddhist herbalists every day. Wild Reishi mushrooms are considered more beneficial than those that are cultivated. Ganoderma Lucidum is composed of carbohydrates, proteins, amino acids, and triterpenoids. The most commonly used Lingzhi mushrooms are the red variety, but all six colors have amazing properties: Red, Black, Green, Purple, Yellow, and White. Lingzhi Mushroom offers some astounding proven health benefits and here are some of them:

Proven Lingzhi Mushroom Benefits:

An Immune System Booster:

Long-term use has proven to be very useful when it comes to strengthening the immune system. Researchers show that polysaccharide beta-1,3-D-glucan in Lingzhi boosts the immune system by raising the number of macrophage T-cells. That's why is recommended for people with AIDS and other immune system disorders.

A Natural Blood Thinner

Lingzhi mushrooms can be used as natural blood thinners instead of aspirin. Reishi mushrooms contain adenosine, a substance that could inhibit blood platelets from sticking together and forming clots. That is good for those with high blood pressure but not for everyone. Also, be careful to not consume Reishi mushrooms if you are taking blood thinners tablets.

Anti-tumor and Anti-cancer Effects of Ganoderma:

Polysaccharides together with triterpenoids are immune-modulating substances and there are defend the DNA and stop cell mutations while protecting the healthy cells.

Liver Protection:

A lot of studies have been published on the usage of Ganoderma in liver protection. Reishi mushroom was able to reduce hepatic injury induced by CCl4.

Helps with Heart Disease:

Studies confirm that Lingzhi mushroom can effectively dilate the coronary artery, improve coronary vessel blood flow, and as a result, is strengthen cardiac muscles!

Neuroprotective Protection:

A Neuropharmacology study made in 2012 shows therapeutic effects on neurodegenerative disorders such as Alzheimer's and Huntington's disease.

Improving Allergies and Asthma:

Ganoderma has a healing effect on the lungs. According to studies in mice and humans, Lingzhi is an expectorant that helps clear mucus from the lungs.

Shimeji Mushrooms:

Shimeji is a food that I frequently order in Japanese restaurants. This mushroom is native to East Asia. Shimeji is a group of edible mushrooms with more than 20 varieties and has a lot of health benefits. These mushrooms can low cholesterol, are good for Weight loss and diabetes management, and have antimicrobial, antiparasitic, and anti-inflammatory properties.

Lion's Mane Mushrooms:

Lion's mane mushrooms are also known as yamabushitake, and Monkey Head mushrooms. It is a saprophytic fungus that is often found on rotten trees in Western Canada, Europe, East Asia, and North America. This mushroom has some very important health benefits, especially for the brain and gut. Studies have shown that the lion's mane contains hericenones and erinacines two special compounds that can stimulate the growth of brain cells and can be able to speed the recovery of minor brain injuries. Another benefit is that it can relieve the symptoms of Depression and Anxiety.

Chaga Mushrooms:

It's called the king of medicinal mushrooms, as it is a super powerful source of nutrients and antioxidants. This fungus is typically found on birch trees. Chaga mushrooms are mainly used to treat tumors, are an immune system booster, slow the aging process, lowering cholesterol, blood pressure, and blood sugar.

Turkey Tail Mushrooms:

The turkey tail is a bracket fungus that grows in tree trunks and deadwood. In Asia, it symbolizes longevity. Turkey tail mushroom has a lot of medicinal properties, is packed with antioxidants, and is famous for its ability to enhance the health of your immune system. It's also useful for fighting certain cancers and for gut bacteria balance.

Cordyceps Mushrooms:

This Chinese medicinal mushroom is known as one of the most effective athletic performance boosters. The spores of Cordyceps fungi are landing, infecting, and killing insects. The roots of the mushroom (Mycelia) begin to grow in the insect, slowly devouring it from the inside. The antioxidant and anti-inflammatory benefits of cordyceps are used for centuries in traditional Chinese medicine. There are 400 species of cordyceps, but Cordyceps Sinensis can be found in the Himalayan foothills of Tibet and Bhutan. Cordyceps can protect against many health diseases like fatigue, depression, asthma and upper respiratory tract infections, diabetes, high cholesterol, kidney disorders, nighttime urination, and male sexual problems.

Portobello Mushrooms:

This Mushroom has a strong, umami flavor that makes them perfect for BBQ and a great alternative to meat. These medicinal mushrooms are known as cancer fighters and immune system protectors. They are high in selenium, copper, potassium, and niacin.

Maitake Mushrooms:

Maitake fungus is among the world's most beneficial mushrooms and has been used as food and medicine in Asia for thousands of years. This fungus offers a wide range of health benefits including its ability to relieve some of the side effects of chemical treatment (chemotherapy) for cancer. It is also used for chronic fatigue syndrome, Polycystic ovary syndrome, HIV/AIDS, hepatitis, Cancer growth, hay fever, high blood pressure, diabetes, high cholesterol, and weight loss.

Chanterelle Mushrooms:

The Chanterelle edible mushroom is a yellow-orange fungus that is delicious and also medicinal. The name Cantharellus is derived from the Greek word 'kantharos' which means clear. Is rich in vitamin D2, vitamin A, vitamin B3 (Niacin), vitamin B5, copper, fatty acids, eight essential amino acids, manganese, and potassium. Chanterelle mushroom improves immune function, is good for the prevention of cardiovascular diseases, reduces the risk of prostate cancer, and is good for bone health.

Truffle Mushrooms:

Truffles are fungi that grow near the roots of specific trees, they have a strong flavor and are a great source of antioxidants. The most important health benefit of Truffles is that promotes "bliss". Apart from that, truffles reduce inflammation, reduce oxidative stress, protect the liver from damage, and might slow down the aging process.

Agarikon Mushrooms:

The ancient Greek physician Dioscorides was named Agarikon mushroom, "elixirium ad longam vitam," which means the elixir of long life. These slow-growing mushrooms are incredibly rare. The Native Americans Shamans believed that Agarikon may give protection against supernatural diseases. Agarikon has many health benefits, this fungus is a strong antibacterial, antiviral and anti-inflammatory agent. Can treat Tuberculosis, Herpes, and certain respiratory problems.

Poria Mushrooms:

It's known as Fu Ling in China and has been used for 2,000 years in traditional Chinese medicine. Poria mushroom contains chemicals that may help fight cancer, Alzheimer's disease, and kidney disease, as well as reduce inflammation, promote sleep, and suppress immune function.

Honey as Medicine:

Honey is well known from ancient times as a food and medicine. Honey has antioxidant, antibacterial, and anti-inflammatory properties. People used honey as an internal and external remedy in ancient Greece, Egypt, and Rome, but also in traditional Chinese medicine and Ayurveda. Studies today have shown that honey has the power to kill bacteria (E. coli, salmonella, H. pylori, etc.)

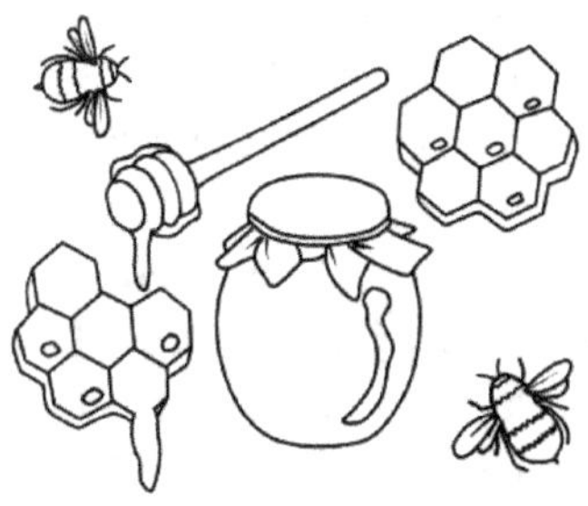

As I mentioned before, the Mediterranean region has very good quality honey, an example is the Elvish honey that costs more than gold. Also, research made on which Greek honey was highest in antioxidant levels has shown that oak honey was the number one, followed by fir honey, reiki honey, chestnut honey, pine honey, thyme honey, and orange honey. Manuka and the Malaysian Tualang honey are also some of the bests in the world. There are so many different types of honey out there like the Acacia Honey, Alfalfa Honey, Aster Honey, Avocado Honey, Basswood Honey, Beechwood Honey, Blueberry Honey, Bluegum Honey, Thyme Honey, Pine Honey, Sage Honey, Sourwood Honey, Tupelo Honey, and the list goes on...

Honeycomb: Propolis, Beeswax,
Bee-pollen, and Royal Jelly:

Honeybees' products have numerous substances, including propolis, beeswax, bee pollen, and royal jelly. Honeycomb is a unique substance and has several benefits to the human body. Honeycombs are commonly found in health food shops. The health benefits of Honeycomb are related to honey, propolis, beeswax, royal jelly, and bee pollen. Honeycomb is a good treatment for allergies, hay fever, and asthma. By chewing honeycomb, you can get rid of headaches, sore throats, and stuffy noses. I love the taste of honeycomb, I chew it like gum until all the honey is out and only pure wax left.

Propolis:

Propolis is the glue of the Bees. It supports the immune system in various ways. Bees create propolis from the resin of trees. It is a mix of beeswax and other secretions. Research and studies showed that propolis may be useful in treating different types of infections. ***Propolis Health Benefits:*** It prevents oral infections, can treats allergies, it's an effective treatment for warts, lowers blood pressure, and may kill colon cancer stem cells.

Bee Pollen:

Bee Pollen is considered one of nature's most completely nourishing foods as it has approximately 40% proteins, vitamins, folic acid, and free amino acids. Actually, pollen has more proteins than any animal source! ***Bee Pollen Benefits:*** Is an energy booster that can help to prevent the onset of asthma. It can be used to treat allergies, boost the immune system, and help the cardiovascular system.

Beeswax:

Beeswax is the main substance of honeycomb, and is comprised largely of fatty acids, hydrocarbons, and esters. I used it in many skin homemade products as it is the best for protecting the skin from environmental toxins and irritants. There are three main types of Beeswax: Yellow, White, and Absolute. *Beeswax Health Benefits:* Beeswax is a great choice for many skin conditions including Dermatitis, Psoriasis, and Eczema. Beeswax protects the liver and lowers the cholesterol levels.

Royal Jelly:

Royal jelly is an ancient remedy. This milky-white secretion is produced by female worker bees and has remarkable antibacterial properties. As royal jelly is exclusive nourishment for bee queens, for humans, is a natural supplement that may provide antibacterial, antioxidant, and anti-inflammatory benefits. *Royal Jelly Health Benefits:* Reduces PMS symptoms and blood sugar levels, can promote fertility, aids in wound healing, can increase testosterone levels, is beneficial to mental health, reduces anemia, boosts immunity and fights infections, reduces allergic reactions, and finally, protects the liver.

I can't write about every type of honey available, so I'll focus on one of the simplest, the Longan flower honey, and one of the most expensive, the Manuka honey.

Longan Flower Honey:

Longan honey is 100% pure raw natural honey. This honey is made from the Longan orchard in the north of Thailand. It is raw, organic, and chemical-free. The longan raw honey consists of active enzymes and natural nutrients. As a result, it can increase and help the absorption of the nutrients in the body, reduce acid in the stomach, reduce fatigue, reduce stress, and improves metabolism. Longan honey has vitamin C, vitamin B, calcium, and phosphorus.

Manuka Honey:

This experiment was made in 2012, and since then, I have treated most of my problems with natural remedies.

Manuka honey is made from the nectar of the manuka tree and is produced only in New Zealand and Australia. Today I buy my first Manuka Honey UMF® 15+. I am the right person to experiment with Manuka as I have some problems with acid reflux, gastritis, and sometimes sinusitis. UMF and MGO are the different ratings available. Ratings on Manuka honey tell you the honey's antibacterial potency. You need at least a Manuka Honey UMF® 15+ to work with H pylori, GERD and Gastritis.

How to Use Manuka Honey for GERD and Gastritis:

Take one teaspoon of this honey four times per day and wait 30 minutes before drinking anything. Do this for the next two weeks.

How to Use Manuka Honey for Sinus Infections:

Mix a cup of distilled hot water with two teaspoons of table salt and propolis (optional). Add one teaspoon of UMF Manuka honey and stir it in until the honey is completely dissolved. Finally, add the liquid to a small spray bottle or a Sterile bottle and spray three times a day or use ten drops of medication into each nostril three times daily.

Manuka Benefits:

It has antibacterial, anti-inflammatory and antioxidant properties. Manuka gives you power and energy and it's an immune system booster. Manuka Honey can treat acid reflux, stomach ulcers, ear or eye infections, sore throat, nasal infections, gastritis, irritable bowel syndrome, ulcerative colitis, and skin-related health problems like Eczema, infections, acne, wounds, burns.

Manuka Honey 7 Days Experiment:

DAY 1) The presence of green mucus indicates that I am infected. I sprayed both nostrils with my manuka bottle and I also ate two teaspoons of Manuka. The flavor is delicious, but I noticed a distinction between Manuka and other types of honey. The flavor was strong, and my throat felt strange. I also felt a slight tingling in my throat, indicating that this Honey is acting as an antibacterial agent.

DAY 2) Today I'm feeling much better, and the green mucus is turning white. I also felt hungrier after eating the honey.

DAY 3) This morning I felt worse and I got a little bit better in the afternoon.

Day 4) The mucus looks cleaner and less. My stomach was a little upset and I had loose stools in the morning…

Day 5) Stools went back to normal. The mucus is cleaner and I didn't have nasal congestion.

Day 6) Today, I feel absolutely fine.

Day Seven and Conclusions:

Manuka honey can likely work as an antibiotic. It helped me to fight the infection at least 70%100. Other things like allergies, LPR, weather conditions, eating habits, and environment are playing also an important role in sinus infection treatment.

Beeswax Vapor Rub and Capsaicin Cream:

Since I have some times allergies and I love sports, I use both Vicks Vapor Rub and Capsaicin Cream. Unfortunately, both of these creams that can be found at pharmacies contain Vaseline. Petroleum jelly (Vaseline) is a mixture of hydrocarbons obtained from petroleum and YES is a toxic risk, as contaminants are linked to cancer. If that is true then why doctors are telling us to use petroleum jelly products on dry skin and eczema and why today it is most commonly used as an ingredient in many cosmetics, lotions, and baby-care products? The reason for this is that many so-called doctors simply repeat what they were taught and do not conduct additional research. Big drug corporations are trying so hard and for many years to convince us that products with Petroleum jelly are innocent. On the other hand, beeswax is useful in countless applications, acts as a repellent (such as Vaseline), and protects against external losses and evaporation of skin moisture.

When combined with olive oil, the famous beeswax-salve is created, which is the purest and most beneficial thing for your skin.

The basic recipe is:

One spoonful of beeswax and seven spoons of olive oil. Melt the beeswax in a bain-marie, add the olive oil, and mix until homogeneous. Take the mixture out from the heat and pour it into a sterile jar. Allow it to cool and solidify until is ready for use. Now if you want to do the Beeswax vapor rub or the Capsaicin cream you will need to pour some essential oils before the mixture completely cools.

I use the same recipe for both, the only difference is the last ingredients. For the Capsaicin cream, I add a half teaspoon of chili powder and for the Vicks vapor rub, I pour 10 Drops of Camphor Essential Oil.

Recipe Ingredients:

A Spoon of Beeswax.
7 Spoons of Virgin Olive Oil.
3 Drops of Oregano Essential Oil.
3 Drops of Glove Essential Oil.
7 Drops of Peppermint Essential Oil.
5 Drops of Cinnamon Essential Oil.
5 Drops of Tea Tree Essential Oil.
10 Drops of Eucalyptus Essential Oil.
10 Drops of Camphor Essential Oil for the Vicks Vapor Rub. Or Half Tea-Spoon of Chili Powder for the Capsaicin Cream. (You can add more Chili Powder if you want the Capsaicin cream stronger).

Beeswax Hair Pomade,
Face Cream and Lip Balm:

Beeswax cream is an ancient recipe for beauty and skincare. It is useful in countless applications, from simple hydration, skincare, and chapped lips, to rashes sores, ulcers, burns, and infections. It has antiseptic, anti-inflammatory, and antifungal healing properties. You can apply it all over the body without any limitations. It is very beneficial, easy to manufacture, and costs not so much money. Just remember, little Vitamin E is always desirable for its antioxidant properties and for extending the product.

Wax for Hair:

Most hair gels out there contain alcohol. So, hair wax is far better as remains applicable and has less chance of drying out. Also, the Beeswax hair pomade is handmade from all-natural ingredients and can help your hair look beautiful and grow faster.

Beeswax Face Cream:

Here's how to make an Organic Anti-Aging Face Cream from scratch. The ingredients are the same as in hair pomade and lip balm.

Beeswax Lip Balm:

This is the easiest way to make a Beeswax natural lip balm. This recipe is great for your lips. Especially if your lips are chapped.

Ingredients:
10 drops of VITAMIN E.
Half Tea-Spoon of Honey.
2 Spoons of Beeswax.
7 Spoons of Olive Oil.
6 Spoons of Coconut Oil.
5 Drops of Tea Tree Essential Oil (Optional).
5 Drops of Mastic Gum Essential Oil (Optional).

Preparation:
Heat the oil in a bain-marie, add the wax and once you remove it from heat and cool it add the essential oils. Then put the mixture into a sterilized glass jar and keep the jar in the fridge if it's summer.

Minerals and Herbs for Libido and Testosterone:

Cure erectile dysfunction and increase testosterone naturally rather than with man-made drugs such as Viagra, Cialis, Levitra, etc. Definitely, other factors like age, nutrition, fitness level, and of course being with the right partner when making love are also important. But besides all the above factors, these herbs may help you as they boost libido and testosterone. These herbs are not as strong as human-made drugs and have fewer side effects. So here are the best minerals and herbs for libido and testosterone.

Catuaba Bark:

This bark increases libido and testosterone. Research showed possible mechanisms of action against low libido through dopamine pathways. It also works by promoting blood flow and opening the blood vessels within the body. Tupi and Guarani Indians used for many years for boosting erection.

Maca Root:

Inca warriors consumed Maca before battle to get energy and power. I tried maca for some time to boost my testosterone in my workouts but actually, it doesn't help. It doesn't help with testosterone but it helps with libido. I felt my libido increase a week after. Studies also support that maca is an aphrodisiac and helps with erectile dysfunction.

Suma Root:

Suma root is a secret gym weapon and a strong adaptogenic herb with ergogenic activity. Suma comes from the Amazon rainforest and is known also as Brazilian Ginseng or The Russian Secret. It is widely used in Latin American countries as a herb that treats various diseases. Over the last ten years, the Suma root has become more famous worldwide due to its use by many athletes at the Olympic Games. This root is known among famous athletes for its anabolic activity (without the side effects of steroidal anabolic drugs). Suma can be used also as an aphrodisiac (along with Maka root and Tribulus Terrestris) and as a natural substitute for Viagra. In the Amazonian rainforest, the locals call Suma "para tudo" which means, for everything…

Suma Root Contains:

Vitamins, minerals, trace elements, and 19 amino acids. Magnesium, cobalt, iron, zinc, vitamins A, B-1, B-2, E, K, and pantothenic acid. It contains also germanium, a powerful antioxidant that strengthens the immune system. Allantoin which accelerates cell renewal, phytohormones, sitosterol, and stigmasterol which have beneficial properties for the heart. Finally, it contains beta-ecdysterone, an ergogenic phytochemical structurally similar to testosterone.

Suma Root Dosage:

Doctors and herbalists in Latin America, and northern European countries, prescribe Suma root in cases such as chronic pain, sexual indifference, low energy levels, and hormonal disorders. *Capsules:* Suma recommended dosage is two or three times per day of 500 – 1,000 mg each time.

Suma Powder Form: Take approximately 1 teaspoon two or three times a day.

Suma Root and Testosterone:

How long for Suma-Root to work as a Testosterone booster? There are many studies about Suma root and Testosterone, so here is one. In 30 days of study, Testosterone was higher for mice that drank Suma root enriched water than for mice that drank plain water. Also, no adverse reactions were seen in mice within 30 days of oral intake.

My Experiment:

I bought the root in powder form and took one teaspoon twice a day for a month.

First Week: After a week my body looks leaner, even if I consume more carbs. I think my metabolism burns more calories, but I'm still a skeptic.

Second Week: After two weeks of Suma root I see a sudden boost in libido, but only if I'm with a girl. Also, my sex performance is better than before.

After a Month: After a Month of Suma-root, I saw a small difference in my muscle growth.

Black Galangal:

Krachai Dum is famous in many countries of Southeast Asia as a natural Viagra. It contains substantial amounts of PDE5 inhibitors, which act like Viagra, but without the negative side effects. It is one of the best herbs for erectile dysfunction. Krachai in the Thai language means Kaempferia-Galanga. So, the real translation for this Thai root (Krachaidam) in English is Black Galangal and not Black Ginger! It is an herbaceous plant and belongs to the Zingiberaceae family (Ginger family). Some doctors claim that after Horny Goat Weed, Black Galangal is the most powerful PDE5 inhibitor and research has backed up these claims. It is used in Thai traditional medicine as a natural testosterone booster for erectile dysfunction in males and as a sex drive herb in females. Krachaidam or Black Ginger is available in the market in various product forms. I used it with zinc for better results.

Black Ginger Benefits:

Thai physicians are using black ginger to prevent strokes. This root has anti-plasmodial, anti-inflammatory, anti-allergic, antioxidant, anti-fungal, anti-mycobacterial, and adaptogenic activity. Studies have shown that it improves erectile function and increases sperm density. According to other research, it increases physical fitness performance and muscular endurance. It stops psoriasis flares. It lowers blood glucose levels and improves blood flow. It reduces triglycerides and helps with gastric ulcers. Finally, it is used as a natural antidepressant.

Doses:

Drink twice a day 30 mg of Black Ginger liqueur (without alcohol). Better after wake up and before going to bed.

Ginseng:

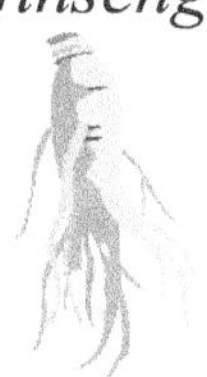

Ginseng is an adaptogen herb and used for a long time in ED treatment. Red ginseng or Panax ginseng is one of the best herbs for Libido. According to studies_nitric oxide relaxes the muscles and promotes blood flow.

Tribulus Terrestris:

Tribulus doesn't help with testosterone problems as some people claim, but yes, it helps with the treatment of erectile dysfunction. Tribulus is most often used for erectile dysfunction, infertility, and low libido. It is known to enhance androgen receptor density in the brain. Studies showed a benefit to people with certain sexual problems and those suffering from infertility. Also, research in Bulgaria and Russia suggested that Tribulus has testosterone-boosting properties. It's a fruit that grows at the base of the leaves. Its a spiny, flat, round, and consists of five seeds. Tribulus thorns inspired the ancient Greeks to construct an insidious weapon that was an iron construction (nails) with four sharp endings, which the ancient Greeks called Tetrahedron.

Tribulus Terrestris Tea:

The herb is harvested without its roots, only the leaves, which have more pronounced properties. Place Tribulus in a pot and cover it with water. Cooked until half of the water is left. The extract is strained and stored in the refrigerator for up to one week. The dosage is three cups of coffee a day (one morning, one afternoon, and the last at night before bed).

Horny Goat Weed:

It is a plant used in traditional Chinese medicine for many years. Epidemium, or Yin Yan Huo in Chinese, is one of the best herbs to treat low libido. Epidemium contains a substance called icariin, which blocks the protein phosphodiesterase type 5 inhibitor (PDE5) which is responsible for low libido in men.

Butea Superba:

Superba is a herb that comes from South East Asia. I saw Butea Superba for the first time in Thailand. Locals used it as an aphrodisiac for many years. Studies have found that is one of the best herbs for men with low libido. Butea Superba has active compounds called cAMP phosphodiesterase inhibitor, that boosts testosterone.

Fenugreek:

Fenugreek or Trigonella is a herb with impressive health benefits. Traditionally it has been used to enhance libido. Recently some studies sawed that it can also boost your testosterone levels. Trigonella has compounds called Furostanolic saponins, which increase testosterone. Also, be careful because Fenugreek can potentially cause gynecomastia.

Ashwagandha:

Ashwagandha is an adaptogen herb that is used in Ayurveda, the traditional medicine of India. This herb can raise sperm quality and testosterone levels. It boosts libido and strengthens the adrenal glands. Finally, another significant benefit of Ashwagandha for men is its anti-anxiety properties.

Boron, Zinc and Selenium:

Boron is a natural element (mineral) that is found in food and the environment. According to a study by NCBI, this mineral increases the metabolism of total testosterone and increases free testosterone levels by nearly 25 percent. As we all know more testosterone equals more sex drive. Zinc and Selenium are also very important for increasing male libido.

Zinc and Selenium help the body produce sex hormones. Together with Boron are some of the best solutions for this problem.

Mucuna Pruriens:

Mucuna Pruriens grows all over India and is an Ayurvedic medicinal herb that increases dopamine. Dopamine influences libido and boosts testosterone. Studies have shown that Mucuna seeds can be used for ED therapy in patients with metabolic diseases.

Tongkat Ali:

I saw Tongkat-Ali (Eurycoma Longifolia) for the first time in Thailand. It is native to Malaysia, lower Burma, Thailand, and Indonesia. Some studies showed that this medicinal plant is shown to increase testosterone and libido in men.

Yohimbe:

Yohimbe comes from the Yohimbe tree. This bark is used a lot in traditional African medicine. The plant has several benefits, but the best is its effect on erectile dysfunction. Many bodybuilding and weight loss supplements contain Yohimbine HCL.

Medicinal Plants for Fever:

Before you search for plants or herbs with antipyretic properties, notice that fever is not your enemy. Fever's purpose is to raise the body's temperature to fight viruses and bacteria. Antipyretics are medicines that lower body temperature when a fever is present. Unfortunately, most of the time those Human-made drugs come with a lot of side effects. Side effects like swelling, hoarseness, hives, difficulty breathing, rash, and itching. As I said above, fever may be a good thing, but in some cases if the fever has gone too high and out of control, then you can use natural medicines to make it go down. So here is a list of the top herbs and plants with Antipyretic activity.

Dong Quai:

It's also called Angelica Sinensis and is native to China, Korea, and Japan. Its root is beneficial for a wide range of ailments, including high blood pressure, anemia, poor circulation, excessive blood sugar, and fever reduction.

Acacia Xanthophloea:

Other names for this plant are Vachellia Xanthophloea or the Fever tree. It is a very popular medicinal plant in Africa and studies have shown that is one of the best plants for treating fevers and eye infections.

Echinacea:

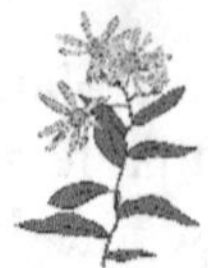

We all know Echinacea as it is recommended by many naturopaths as an immune system booster. Echinacea is used in Europe and North America (by Native Americans) for the treatment of common cold, flu, sore throat, cough, and yes fever. Today studies provide evidence that Native Americans were right.

Yarrow:

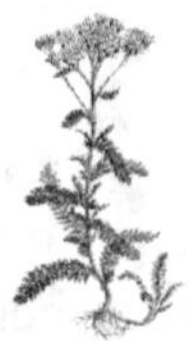

It's one of the best herbs for fever. It is known as yarrow and Achillea millefolium. The name was derived from Achilles, the hero of Greek mythology, who healed his wounds with this plant.

Devil's Claw Root:

A flowering plant of the sesame family. It is native to southern Africa and has been used medicinally for thousands of years. This plant has a lot of health benefits and one of them is that reduces fever.

Tamarind:

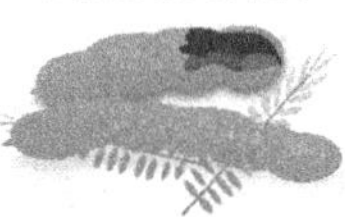

Tamarind has many antioxidant and anti-inflammatory properties. Although native to Africa, this fruit has become one of the most important ingredients of Asian cuisine. Rich in thiamin, iron, magnesium, and phosphorus, it is also recognized for its ability to reduce fever.

Sage:

As a tea, it has antioxidant and anti-inflammatory properties. Sage was considered a sacred herb by the ancient Greeks. Sage tea is effective for relieving your sore throat and has also antipyretic activity.

Lemon Balm:

Is a member of the mint family with anti-viral and anti-stress properties. It is used to treat stomach cramps, headaches, fever, and urinary infections. The ancients Greeks and Romans used lemon balm to treat fevers.

Chilli:

We all know that people eat a lot of chilies in warm countries like Thailand, Mexico, and Indonesia, and there is a reason for this. Capsaicin in chili peppers increases metabolism and can reduce body temperature. Chilli has a strong analgesic and antipyretic effect.

Borage:

Also known as the bee plant or Starflower. It is native to Mediterranean countries and has anti-inflammatory properties. The flower and leaves are good for the treatment of fever, stress, cough, and rheumatoid arthritis.

Ginger:

Try a tea with ginger, honey, and lemon. Ginger has antibacterial, anti-viral properties and is really effective against fever.

Elderflower:

Many people know Elderflower for treating sinusitis, but most importantly elderflower tea can also reduce fever and give wellness to the patient.

Basil:

Basil is native to tropical regions, and it is popular as a food seasoning. As tea is an effective herb for bringing down fever.

Garlic:

Garlic is famous around the world. It is packed with many antibacterial properties and can lower fever by promoting sweating.

Tea Types and their Benefits:

There are so many tea types, different teas with different health benefits. But let's clear something, herbal Teas are actually not teas, as all real teas come from the same plant, the Camellia Sinensis. The real name that we should use is herbal beverages. For example, Chamomile Tea, Peppermint Tea, Ginger Tea, Sage Tea, and so on are all herbal beverages and usually are not contain any caffeine. Now, let's jump to the real different teas and their benefits.

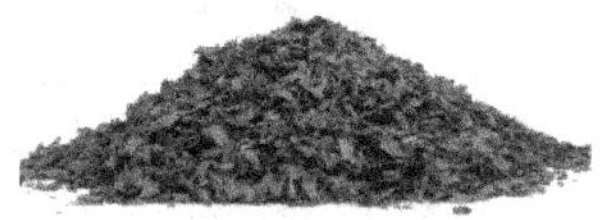

Black Tea:

Black tea is more oxidized than green, oolong, and white teas and blended with other plants for more flavor like earl grey. Dark tea or black tea has less caffeine than coffee but more caffeine than all the other teas. It also contains a lot of antioxidants like polyphenols that block DNA damage. Black tea helps the body metabolize sugar, increases energy, boosts heart health, is good for the bones, and can prevent cancer.

Oolong Tea:

Oolong comes from China and has many similarities with black and green teas. Is a semi-oxidized tea with a lot of health benefits. It helps with losing weight and metabolism, can lower blood sugar levels, is good for the heart, improves brain function, and may protect against certain Cancers.

Green Tea:

We all know green tea and how important is for our health as it contains a lot of Flavonoids like catechins (EGCG) and epicatechins. Green tea may lower harmful LDL cholesterol levels, increase metabolism, and help with weight loss. Regulates glucose levels, protects against the formation of clots, can reduce the risk of cancer, and protects against Alzheimer's and Parkinson's diseases. Finally, this tea boosts your brain and helps with depression.

Matcha Tea:

Matcha is a powerful concentrated ground powder of green tea leaves. The difference is that green tea leaves are the finest and are always harvested by hand. When someone drinks matcha, is consuming the whole tea leaf which has more benefits and is higher in nutrients, and Flavonoids like EGCG catechin, and L-theanine.

White Tea:

The difference with white tea is that it is the least processed. The leaves and buds are picked when they are still young and just before they are fully open. This is also the reason that white tea it's rich in antioxidants and can reduce the risk of heart disease, can help with weight loss, may fight Cancer, improves hair and skin health, has anti-diabetic properties, helps reduce inflammation, improves liver health, and is good for the teeth.

Puer Tea:

Pu-erh tea is the most oxidized form of tea and originates from the Yunnan province of China. This tea can be very expensive as antique Puerh tea is similar to good quality wine. Pu Erh also has lower caffeine content than black tea. This tea can raise the level of good cholesterol (HDL) and lower the level of bad cholesterol (LDL), increases energy, prevents cancer, protects bone health, reduce stress, reduce diabetes and cardiovascular diseases, and promote blood circulation.

Yellow Tea:

We all know black, green, Oolong, and Puer teas, but what about Yellow Tea (huángchá in Chinese)? This little-known tea has a unique taste and remarkable benefits. The process is similar to that of green tea with the only difference being that the leaves are allowed to oxidize more. The benefits of this tea are the same as black and green tea.

Psychoactive Drugs of Mother Nature:

My work as a natural medicine researcher will be incomplete without the "benefits" of psychoactive drugs. The purpose of this chapter is to understand that everything is for a reason in nature. Mother Earth's pharmacy has many mysterious plants. There is a misconception that drugs that occur organically in nature are safe. NO, THEY ARE NOT! Do I believe that some of these drugs have spiritual (open mind) effects? Yes, I do, but without a doubt, most of the time drugs, even from nature, have opposite effects. We all must understand that these psychoactive drugs are very dangerous especially if you don't have a naturopathic doctor or better a Shaman that has the knowledge for any of these drugs and of course the doses. Psychoactive drugs even if found in nature are not good for consumption as they can cause many side effects and even sometimes permanent damage if taken for many years. Also, many of the benefits from those plants can be found in other ways. So, it's mostly a risk to use them. NOTE: I'm responsible for what I write, not for what you understand. This list is only for research purposes, so do not blame me if you are stupid enough to try any of these psychoactive drugs. Now that I clear this, here are the *Top Psychoactive Drugs of Mother Nature*:

Cannabis:

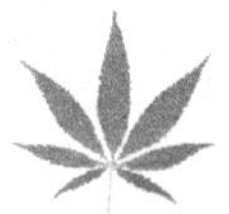

It's one of the most famous psychoactive drugs and is also known as marijuana or weed. THC is the main psychoactive constituent of weed. Today we finally know that CBD (the other prevalent cannabinoid found in cannabis) and THC have many medical benefits. CBD doesn't cause the psychoactive effects that occur on THC. Cannabis today is used to treat many diseases including seizures, IBS, inflammation, depression, migraines, anxiety, insomnia, Multiple sclerosis, Parkinson's disease, muscle spasms, Alzheimer's disease, low appetite, glaucoma, PTS disorder, and even cancer.

Magic Mushrooms:

Psilocybin is a naturally occurring psychedelic compound. There are about two hundred different species of magic mushrooms. These mushrooms are sometimes used as a medicine to treat some really bad disorders including anxiety, cluster headaches, depression, and OCD. Magic Mushrooms have a lot of dangers. Even with low dosages, you can get a psychotic episode and suffer from temporary paranoia. Psilocybin was banned in 1970, and after 30 years of suspension, it's again allowed for research purposes. Magic mushroom's health benefits and healing effects are both medical and psychological.

Magic Mushrooms Health Benefits:

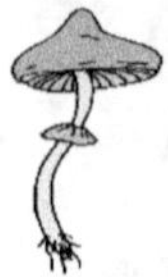

Stimulates Growth of New Brain Cells:
Research showed that psilocybin helps mice promote new neurons growth and regeneration in their brains.

Treating Depression:
A study from Imperial College London found that magic mushrooms were very effective for treating depression, with 5 of 12 being completely cured of their depression and the rest experiencing a major reduction in depression symptoms.

Alleviates Obsessive-Compulsive Disorder Symptoms:
Studies showed that psilocybin mushrooms are effective at reducing the symptoms of OCD.

Psilocybin as a Treatment for a Cluster Headache:
Cluster headache sufferers and researchers found that small doses of Psilocybin can end cluster headache cycles and prevent entire cycles from starting.

Psilocybin Dosages:
Low doses don't produce the "bad trip" effect and can offer long-term benefits. By taking low doses, we have a very low possibility of a significant fear reaction. So low dosage that is not more than 10 mg with a doctor control. NOTE: Please for safety reasons, do not take any doses of Psilocybin without a doctor.

Morning Glory:

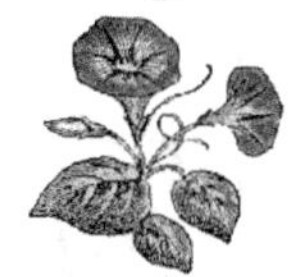

Morning glory seeds are called Tlitlitzin and contain an intoxicating chemical similar to LSD. Were used ritually by the Aztec Shamans for their psychoactive properties. This powerful hallucinogenic compound of Morning glory seeds is often referred to as LSA. The plant is an adaptogen. The calming effect of this flower alleviates the symptoms of stress. This large family comprises over a thousand flowering plant species.

Hawaiian Baby Woodrose:

Hawaiian Baby Woodrose is a member of the Morning Glory family and contains A tryptamine called LSA (Lysergic Acid Amide). As mentioned before this compound has a long shamanic history. This plant creates strong psychedelic experiences. In Indian Ayurvedic medicine, it is used to treat rheumatism, elephantiasis, and inflammation of the joints.

Sassafras Plant:

Sassafras was used for flavoring root beer. Safrole can be used to make either MDA or MDMA (ecstasy). The FDA banned sassafras in 1979, not only for the psychoactive compounds found in the plant but also because research showed it caused cancer in rats. Other studies showed that sassafras in small doses can treat cancer. Sassafras is used to treat arthritis, bronchitis, urinary tract disorders, gout, syphilis, high blood pressure, skin problems, and even cancer. MDMA is synthetic drug-using safrole as its main ingredient.

MDMA was a drug made by the FDA, and it was used as psychotherapy to treat patients with psychiatric disorders.

Angel's Trumpets:

The leaves and flowers of the plant are used to make medicine and it has been used in India for centuries in Ayurvedic medicine. It's poisonous and eating the flower can give you hallucinations and euphoria, but also it can leave you dead. Psychoactive compounds of the plant are known chemically as tropane alkaloids. the leaves of Angel's Trumpets can use for asthma treatment.

Opium Poppies:

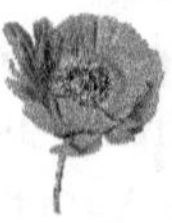

Opium is the main source of morphine and codeine, the two most commonly used analgesic painkillers. This flower has been used as medicine for centuries. Heroin comes from the dried latex of opium poppies. Bayer, in the 1890s, promoted heroin for use in children suffering from colds. This product is called heroin and supposedly makes you 'heroic'. Opium causes euphoria and peacefulness but can also create memory problems, confusion, convulsions, and hallucinations.

Coca Plant – Cocaine:

When I was in Peru and Bolivia, I saw people chew coca leaves just to relieve hunger and to enhance physical performance. Coca leaves are also used as a painkiller and for reducing the unwanted symptoms of altitude sickness. As tea is great medicine for an upset stomach and Asthma. For Incas coca was a sacred plant with magical powers. It is said that

Incas may have been using coca leaves compounds like a liquid to perform brain surgery 3,500 years ago. Cocaine is a drug extracted from coca plant leaves in powder form.

Tobacco (Nicotianatabacum):

According to a study funded in part by NIDA Nicotine may not be the only psychoactive component in tobacco smoke. We all know that smoking is one of the worst things you can do for your health, but even Tobacco is there for a reason. If smoking is moderate (even if it seems almost impossible), some benefits are: Smoking alleviates ulcerative colitis and protects against Parkinson's Disease. Nicotine can enhance brain function in people with cognitive decline. Smoking lowers the risk of obesity and helps with depression. Nicotine creates an immediate sense of relaxation.

Caffeine-Plants:

Coffee, tea, yerba maté, guarana, kola nut, cacao, and more. Caffeine is the world's most famous psychoactive substance. It is an alkaloid that exists naturally in more than 60 plant species. In moderation, caffeine has a lot of health benefits. Caffeine improves energy levels and relieves post-workout muscle pain by up to 48%. Can help you burn fat, and may protect against Parkinson's disease and Dementia. May lower your risk of type 2 diabetes and it increases stamina during exercise. Caffeine may reduce fatty liver, and works as a bronchodilator in patients with asthma. Finally, it is good for the heart and can fight depression.

Ethanol Sources:

Ethanol is naturally produced by fermentation. Fermentation is a biological process. Alcohol can be produced from many natural sources, including corn, bagasse, wheat, miscanthus, switchgrass, grain sorghum, barley, potatoes, hemp, cassava, kenaf, and sunflower. Also, sugar crops such as sugar cane, sugar beet, and sweet sorghum. Ethanol is a psychoactive substance and is the active ingredient in all Alcoholic Beverages. Moderate alcohol consumption may provide some health benefits: Can lower the risk of cardiovascular disease, can decrease the chances of developing dementia, boosts your brainpower, reduces the risk of gallstones, and makes you happy.

Datura Plants:

Datura contains 10 to 12 species of flowering plants. These plants are used in magic and shamanic rituals but also for medical purposes. The Datura plants contain the highest number of toxic alkaloids and can be even fatal. Are often confused with angels' trumpets, but angels' trumpets are related to the genus Brugmansia. In Ayurveda medicine, is used to treat fever, bronchitis and asthma, inflammations, and mental disorders.

Mescaline Cactuses:

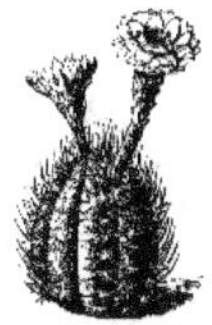

Mescaline is a natural psychedelic alkaloid found in cacti like San Pedro cactus, Bolivian torch, and Peyote (Lophophora williamsii). Peyote is native to the deserts of southern Texas and Mexico. The Native American tribes Navajo, Lipan Apache, Tonkawa, and Mescalero used Mescaline for spiritual experiences and medicinal purposes. Mescaline is also used for the treatment of alcoholism, pain, and depression. Finally, in an experiment with Human subjects' mescaline promoted growth hormone levels.

Ephedra Plant:

Ephedra is a herb that has been used in Traditional Chinese Medicine for more than 5,000 years. Ephedra plant contains the alkaloids ephedrine and pseudoephedrine, the principal chemicals for Methamphetamine. Bodybuilders use many times ephedra as a fat-burning supplement. It is also used for allergies, nasal congestion, asthma, and bronchitis.

Wormwood Artemisia Absinthium:

Wormwood has psychoactive (Thujone) and hallucinogenic properties. The traditional absinthe is made of fennel, anise, and of course wormwood. The Egyptians and the Greeks used the herb in their traditional medicines. Wormwood has long been used to kill parasites but also to treat gall bladder disease, fever, liver disease, sexual desire, depression, memory loss, and muscle pain.

Kratom Plant:

Kratom is a tropical tree with leaves that have psychotropic properties and is native to Southeast Asia. Most of the time people in southeast Asia chew kratom leaves, but they can also be crushed and smoked or brewed into tea. Here are some health benefits of kratom leaves in lower doses. Kratom is an immune system booster, a pain reliever, a sexual stimulant, reduces anxiety, and is good for diabetes management. A study showed that using kratom can treat post-traumatic stress disorder and social anxiety.

Salvia Divinorum Plant:

Salvia Divinorum is another plant with psychoactive hallucinogenic properties and like Kratom, the leaves are consumed by chewing, smoking, or as a tea. It is still used by the Mazatec tribe, to create shamanic visions for healing purposes. As a medicine, Salvia can reduce depression and anxiety, relieve chronic pain, and can help to manage issues like diarrhea, upset stomach, headaches, anemia, and rheumatism.

Ayahuasca Plants:

Ayahuasca is an ancient psychoactive brew made from the Banisteriopsis caapi vine and the Psychotria Viridis leaf. It's called sacred plant medicine. Many tribes of Amazonia say that Ayahuasca is a portal and can heal the mind, body, and spirit within the past, present, and future. Only experienced shamans can lead you on this healing trip. Banisteriopsis caapi "the vine of the soul" is a hallucinogenic vine in the Malpighiaceae plant family. The three main alkaloids (harmala alkaloids) in Banisteriopsis caapi are Harmine, tetrahydroharmine, and harmaline. Banisteriopsis caapi is a great antioxidant and a brain enhancer, it may protect against Parkinson's Disease and can help with depression and anxiety.

Psychotria Viridis leaf also is known as Chacruna. It contains a high concentration of a natural psychoactive compound called DMT. Psychotria Viridis leaf can help to vomit to expel infectious parasites and bacteria. DMT also demonstrated a marked activity against tumor cell strains. Finally, Psychotria Viridis leaf is also very helpful with lung infections and colds. In general, Ayahuasca cures cancer, and PTSD, clears the Body from Parasites, reduces depression, and most important Ayahuasca has inner self-healing benefits, as it expands consciousness.

Mad honey:

Mad honey is made by bees that feed on rhododendron flowers that contain grayanotoxins. Grayanotoxins have hallucinogenic properties and some medicinal benefits. In Nepal and Turkey, mad honey is used as an aphrodisiac, as a medicine, as a drug, and even as a biological weapon during war. As medicine was used to treat diabetes, arthritis, hypertension, libido, and stomach diseases.

Mandrake root:

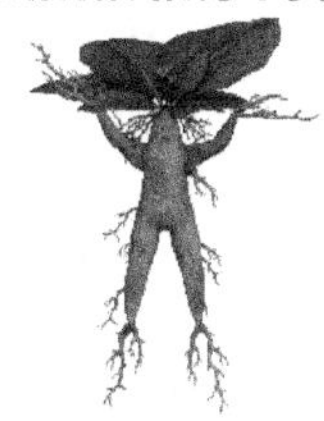

Mandrake root (Mandragora) has an anthropomorphic shape and that's why people were always curious about this plant. In the Mediterranean and the Middle East was used for sorcery and as herbal medicine. The Greek doctor Dioscorides, tells us that mandrake root was used in ancient

Rome as an anesthetic, hallucinogen, painkiller, and aphrodisiac. Today Mandrake root, especially European mandrake root used for treating asthma, constipation, stomach ulcers, hay fever, and rheumatism.

Betel Nut:

They say that is like a combination of tobacco with a lot of caffeine, but people who chew Betel Nut because of its CNS stimulating effects get really high. It's very popular in Southeast and South Asia. As a traditional medicine, it increased stamina, boosts appetite, helps with eye care, and is euphoric. Betel Nut detoxifies the body and helps with flatulence or constipation, and finally can help with stroke recovery.

Belladonna Plant:

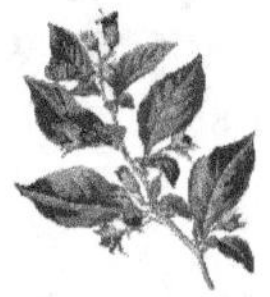

Do you remember the belladonna song from the UFO band in 1976? Yes, the song was not about the beautiful (Bella) Dona, but about a plant that causes wild hallucinations and is used as a poison. Atropa belladonna is used to treat tremors, Parkinson's disease, nerve problems, hay fever, arthritis, asthma, motion sickness, nausea, and vomiting.

Best Herbs for Liver Cleansing:

The liver is the largest gland and largest abdominal organ in the body and is protected by the rib cage. The liver creates proteins, manufactures, and regulates hormones, changing food into energy and cleaning toxins from the blood. Unfortunately, many different diseases can occur in the liver like fatty liver, hepatitis, cirrhosis, gallstones, non-alcoholic fatty liver disease, etc. Fatty foods and alcohol can be toxic to the liver (hepatotoxic), especially in high doses.

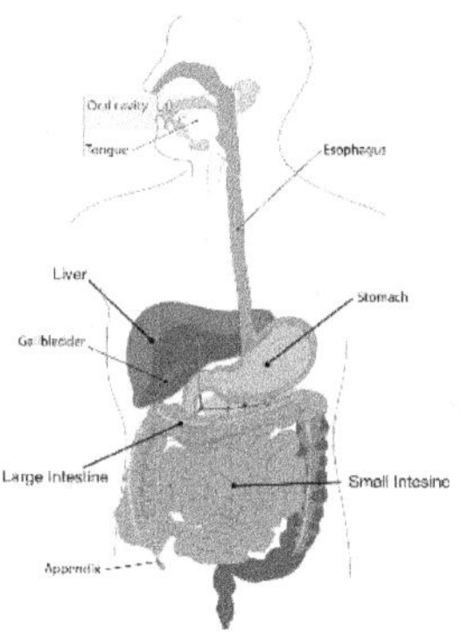

Signs and symptoms of liver disease:
Abdominal pain, loss of appetite, diarrhea, yellowing of the skin and whites of the eyes, a high-temperature fever, itchy skin, weight loss, and swelling in the legs and feet. If you detox your liver, you detox your whole body, but which are the herbs for liver protection? Fortunately, many herbs can help with liver cleansing. One thing to remember is that all herbs that detoxify the liver are bitter.

Liver Detox Herbs:

Artichoke:

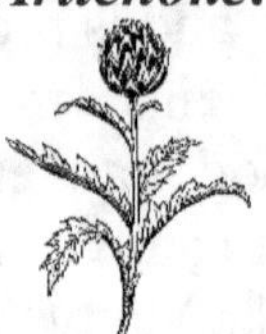

Artichoke is one of my favorite plants and one of the best herbs for the Liver. Believe it or not, Artichokes are actually flower buds. This bitter plant contains potent antioxidants and prebiotics. Artichoke is good for gut flora, detoxification, and weight loss. European doctors, naturopaths, and holistic doctors are prescribing artichoke extracts to those with liver problems for many years now. Artichoke contains luteolin, niacin, caffeoylquinic acid, iron, phosphorus, chlorogenic acid, apigenin, sterols, vitamin C, vitamin B6, vitamin K, potassium, copper, folic acid, magnesium, fiber, inulin, and polyphenols.

Milk Thistle:

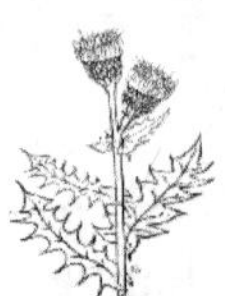

I saw Milk Thistle for the first time in my village in Greece. People use milk thistle as medicine for more than 2,000 years. This flower protects your liver and has an antioxidant and free radical scavenging action. Silymarin is the main active ingredient in milk thistle, which is extracted from the plant's seeds.

Turmeric:

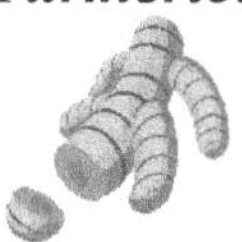

This spice is medicine. It is used mostly for liver disease, skin problems, and gastrointestinal problems. An animal study showed that curcumin reduces liver damage. Turmeric contains minerals like calcium, potassium, iron, manganese, zinc, copper, and magnesium. Also, components including beta-carotene, vitamin C, Vitamin B-6, flavonoids, fiber, and niacin.

Dandelion:

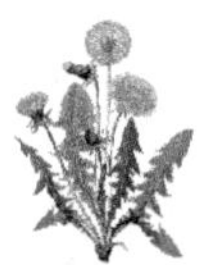

Taraxacum is a flower native to Europe and North America. It contains vitamin A, vitamin B6, vitamin C, vitamin K and minerals like iron, magnesium, calcium, potassium, and sodium. Many people use the bitter dandelion root to detoxify, clean the liver, and promote increased bile production. Research from the Journal of Medicinal Food shows that dandelion helps to protect the liver from drugs, including painkillers that cause serious liver damage in high doses like acetaminophen

Cardamom:

Originated in India, is an expensive spice found in the form of a small pod that inside has black seeds with impressive medicinal properties. Cardamom is rich in potassium, magnesium, calcium, phosphorus, vitamin C, fiber, pyridoxine, sodium, iron, zinc, and vitamin B like thiamin, riboflavin, niacin, and vitamin B6. The seeds of Cardamom are great for liver cleansing and detox.

Foods that can Prevent Sugar Spikes:

We all need foods that can prevent sugar spikes. Normally carbs are what cause blood sugar to rise as they are broken down into simple sugars within our body. Our pancreas releases insulin hormone that converts food into energy. If insulin is out of balance, we have a problem called insulin resistance that can lead to elevated cortisol. Cortisol is a steroid stress hormone secreted by the adrenal glands and turns energy into fat. Both of these hormones (insulin and cortisol) are extremely useful, but when they are out of balance, they can cause stress and weight problems.

Baobab Fruit:

This fruit is rich in vitamins and minerals like vitamin C, vitamin B6, antioxidants, niacin, magnesium, potassium, calcium, iron, and zinc. Studies showed that this African fruit regulates blood sugar and decreased the amount of insulin. It is also one of the best prebiotics out there. Yes, Baobab is the superfruit of Africa's 'Tree of Life'.

Apple Cider Vinegar:

We all know the power of apple cider vinegar for acid reflux and GERD, but what we don't know is that it lowers blood sugar and insulin spikes during a high-carb meal by 19–34%. One or two teaspoons before or with meals are the recommended doses to boost weight loss and help with insulin resistance and blood sugar.

Cinnamon:

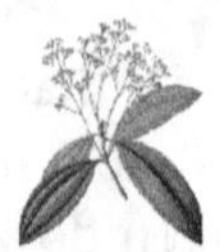

Cinnamon is one of the best friends of sugar. We all love this combination. Honey and Cinnamon are some of the best combos as both have a lot of antioxidants and healing properties. Now, what most people don't know is that according to studies, cinnamon increases insulin sensitivity in people and lowers blood sugar levels.

Bitter Melon:

I tasted a bitter melon for the first time in South East Asia and believe me it was not pleasant at all. This vegetable has many health benefits. A lot of studies have shown that bitter melon has properties that act like insulin and help to lower blood sugar levels.

Green Tea:

Green tea is gaining popularity as is one of the healthiest beverages out there. A lot of studies and research have shown that green tea and especially Japanese matcha tea reduces insulin resistance and improves glycemic control.

Fatty Fish:

Oily fish are the best sources of omega-3s. A study showed that omega-3 fatty acids are associated with increased insulin sensitivity. Fish like salmon, mackerel, Sardines, Tuna, Striped bass, Perch, and so on. Individuals with a higher omega-3 index have a lower risk of type 2 diabetes.

Cacao:

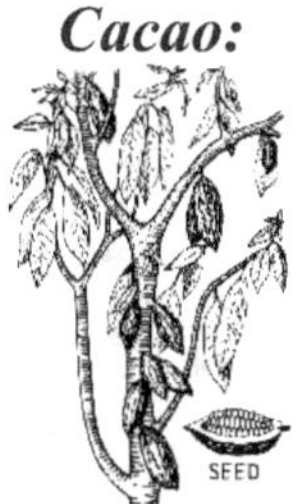

Cacao is another Super-food that helps with sugar spikes. According to studies, consumption of dark chocolate rich in flavanol has been shown to decrease blood pressure and insulin resistance.

Natural Antibiotics:

The purpose of common antibiotics is to eliminate germs, but here is the problem, not all bacteria are dangerous, and some may be necessary for our body. Common antibiotics kill both good and bad bacteria. Natural antibiotics, on the other hand, work in two primary ways. first, they eliminate dangerous germs, and second, they boost the body's defenses. It is all here, nature has effective substances with natural antiviral and antibacterial properties.

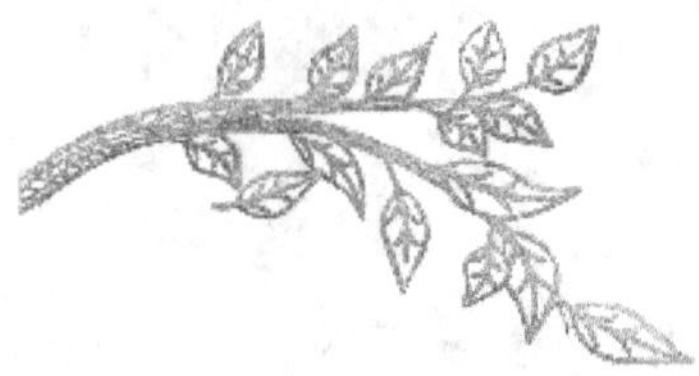

Garlic Clove:

Garlic is one of the best natural antibiotics. Over the years, garlic has been used as a medicine to treat many different diseases. Take three to five cloves a day if you have a strong stomach or 600 to 1000 mg of garlic extract daily.

Vitamin C:

Vitamin C is one of the top natural antibiotics. Did you know that some animals can make their own vitamin C, but people can't? No problem at all, as we can find Vitamin C in many fruits and vegetables.

Echinacea:

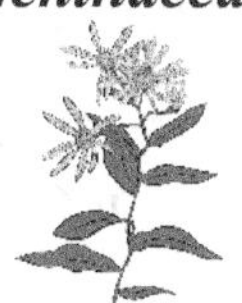

Echinacea is very popular for the treatment of flu and colds. Originated in eastern North America. Echinacea works similarly to garlic. Native American Indians used the plant in order to combat respiratory infections, toothache, and snake bites.

Pau D'Arco:

Pau d'arco originated in the rainforests of Central and South America. Dried Pau d'Arco can be used as tea. Native American Indians used this herbal medicine with a wide range of health benefits.

Propolis and Good Quality Honey Like Manuka:

Propolis has been used as a traditional medicine for many centuries instead of common antibiotics. Manuka honey is from New Zealand. Bees pollinate the native manuka bush, and new research has shown that manuka honey can eliminate every type of bacteria. Maori tribe was the first to identify the healing properties of manuka honey.

Ginseng:

This root used as a natural antibacterial in Korean and Chinese herbal medicine for thousands of years. Ginseng was also used by many Native American tribes.

Raw Apple Cider Vinegar:

Apple cider vinegar was used by the Greek father of medicine, Hippocrates, to treat many health conditions. He recommended it to his patients for its healing antibiotic properties.

Colloidal Silver:

Colloidal silver is famous as a powerful natural antibiotic against infections. However, some experts think that can be harmful.

Natural Antihistamines for Allergies:

Histamines are released by the body during a time of an allergy attack and stress. An allergic reaction often occurs without no one knowing what causes it. Allergies, in general, are an overreaction of our immune system. Our body confuses a foreign substance (such as pollen, dust mites, or pet dander) as an invader and produces histamines. Histamines play an important role in our body and brain. Allergies can sometimes be a reaction to a particular combination of the foods we eat. So why do we need antihistamines? The antihistamine blocks the histamine from attaching to histamine receptors. One of the benefits of natural antihistamines is that it is much less likely to cause any side effects like antihistamine medications.

We separate allergies into 3 categories:
•Inhalant allergens: House dust mites, mold, pet dander, spores, pollen, etc.
•Ingestant (food) allergens: Milk, eggs, peanuts, fish, certain medications, soy, wheat, etc.
•Contactant allergens: Certain cosmetics and metals such as a watch, necklace, etc.

Foods to Avoid:
Foods made with a large amount of yeast.
Sugar foods.
Aged or fermented cheeses.
Processed meats.

Top Natural Antihistamines:
Basil:
Butterbur:
Butterbur is one of the best and could be an effective herbal treatment for hay fever.
Bromelain:
Helpful for cleaning mucus, making it easier for people to breathe. Bromelain is an extract derived from the stems of pineapples.
Flavonoids:
Colorful fruits and vegetables, blueberries, strawberries, and so on…
Parsley, Cardamom, Ginger, Chamomile, Fennel:
Quercetin (Found in wine and many fruits and vegetables).
Stinging Nettle:
Thyme:
Omega-3 Fatty Acids:
Their anti-inflammatory properties reduce allergic reactions.

NATURAL TREATMENTS

Information about all kinds of natural treatments that can support your health. We focus on the value of good health and general well-being. Before starting any therapies, we must locate the source of the issue in order to treat symptoms and illnesses. Natural medicines, complementary alternative therapies, and integrative therapies are all included in a holistic healthcare approach.

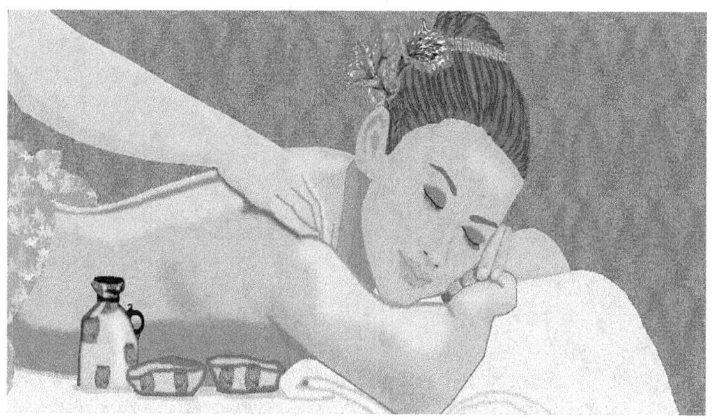

Crying and Laughter Health Benefits:

Humans have so many feelings, but crying and laughing are, without a doubt, two very strong emotions that also have numerous health benefits. Increased emotions, like laughing and crying are very close. We can all laugh to a point of tears. But the most important benefit for me with both crying and laughing is that we free our feelings.

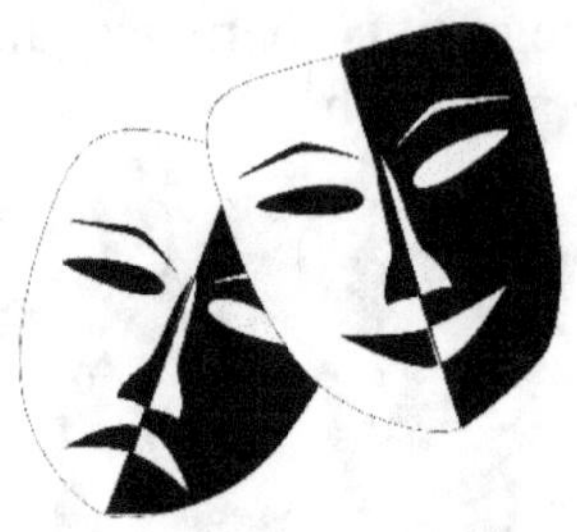

Crying and Health:

Strong emotions like rage, grief, sadness, frustration, and joy come with crying. Crying has healing and detoxifying powers. Studies have shown that crying is good for both body and mind. Just remember, at birth, the baby's first cry is a sign that the baby is healthy. Japanese believe in the health benefits of crying so much that now have the so-called crying clubs (rui-katsu).

Crying Health Benefits:

It Helps Release Stress:
We all know that crying is taking out our negative emotions.

Crying Relieves Pain:
Studies showed that chemicals like oxytocin and endorphins are released with crying which helps relieve pain.

It Helps with Insomnia:
As it helps with stress and negativity, crying is reduced insomnia.

Crying Restores Emotional Balance:
This is one of my favorites, as emotional balance is very important for general wellness and bliss.

Improves Vision:
Crying helps our eyes to cleanse themselves.

Crying Cleanses the Lymphatic System:
Believe it or not, a good cry can clean your lymphatic system. Tears help the body to get rid of the toxins and chemicals that raise cortisol.

Laughter and Health:
Some say that laughter is the best medicine, and I agree if combined with a healthy diet and regular exercise. Healthy laughter triggers endorphins and releases emotions like relief, joy, happiness, fan, and so on. Laughing clubs and laughter yoga (Hasyayoga) are very good for health.

Laughter Health Benefits:

It Helps Release Stress:
Laughter shuts down the release of stress hormones like cortisol.

Laughter Lowers Blood Pressure:
Studies found that laughter can lower your blood pressure levels.

It Burns Calories:
Studies showed that laughing for 15 minutes a day can burn about 45 calories.

Is an Immune Booster:
With laughing we activate T-cells that boost our immune system.

Is a Natural Anti-Depressant:
Laughter therapies and studies have shown that laughing reduces depression and helps with mood improvement.

Is Good for the Heart:
Research has shown that laughter is good for our cardiovascular system.

Oil Pulling Therapy:

Oil pulling is the act of swishing oil (Virgin olive oil, Sesame, and Coconut oil recommended) in the mouth for up to 5 or 10 minutes to improve health. Oil pulling is a traditional Indian therapy that dates back over 3,000 years. Our mouth is home to millions of bacteria, fungi, toxins, and viruses and the oil acts as a cleanser.

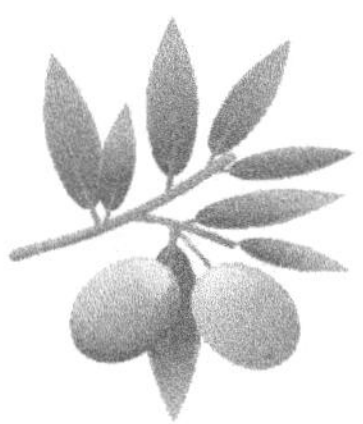

Olive Oil Pulling Benefits:

This ancient treatment has many health benefits. It is a simple but highly effective method. It has proven beneficial for many disorders such as:

Blood diseases.
Lung and liver disorders.
Tooth disease and gum.
Headaches.
Dermatoses.
Peptic ulcers.
Intestinal disorders.
Lack of appetite.
Heart disease and kidney.
Encephalitis.
Neurological problems.
Poor memory.

All you have to do is to keep the oil in your mouth for a few minutes. The olive oil will be mixed with the saliva and it will activate enzymes that attract toxins from the blood. That's why it is important to keep the oil for at least five minutes before you spit it. After five minutes you will realize that the oil becomes milky white or yellow color since it is saturated by toxins and harmful bacteria! In the end, rinse your mouth with a half teaspoon of baking soda or with natural sea salt. The baking soda or the natural sea salt removes the oil residues and toxins.

COVID-19 Natural Treatment:

My Journal on Covid:

After the bird flu in 2005, here I'm again in Asia with another Pandemic disease, Coronavirus-COVID-19. Headache, running nose, cough, sore throat, loss of smell (anosmia) or taste, fever, and even lethargy are the COVID-19 Symptoms in Humans. Similar to flu and upper respiratory tract infections. A pandemic is an epidemic disease that spreads across a wide geographical area and affects all of humanity. Fortunately, I'm not in China where coronavirus started, but I'm in a place with a lot of Chinese tourists, Thailand. Bangkok and other big cities in Thailand look like hospitals, as so many people wear those white surgical masks. I'm also wearing one, the terrible news spread so quickly thanks to media reports, who wants to get sick after all? But is raising awareness or creating fear? Or is it just a new way for big pharma to profit from vaccines? Where is Ebola today, and what about the mad cow or bird flu diseases? Two potential diseases that impacted the world economy. Vaccines are a multibillion-dollar industry.

Coronavirus is a zoonotic disease that is transmitted from animals to humans. For example, bats or snakes may pass it to humans. But wait, Chinese people, eating these animals for over two thousand years, so why now? Why did this disease come just before the Chinese New Year, the time that the Chinese traveled all around the world? Also, why don't we see coronavirus infections in animals? Yes, coronaviruses are a family of viruses, and it is maybe a coincidence that in 2004, the CDC filed a patent on a newly isolated coronavirus known as SARS, and expired on January 24, 2020. Also in 2015, the Pirbright Institute filed a patent for a live attenuated coronavirus to be used in the production of vaccines.

An emergent virus is a virus that has adapted and emerged as a new disease. The book Emerging Viruses AIDS and Ebola by Harvard researcher Leonard G. Horowitz gathers evidence that HIV and Ebola were laboratory creations that were transmitted into the general population by vaccine experiments of hepatitis, polio, and smallpox. I don't want to believe that these dark-side people exist and that are capable of killing so many people just for profit. Anyway, nobody knows what will happen with Coronavirus tomorrow. We also don't know how many other Epidemic-Pandemic Diseases will happen in the future.

Now a year later, my journal for this deadly virus continues. From Thailand, I'm back in Greece now. COVID-19 spreads outside Asia, and countries like Italy, Germany, and England, are leading the world with new coronavirus cases. So, as COVID-19 crackdowns grow in Europe, the EU closes borders to slow down COVID-19. Every day, we learn something new about the virus that continues to frighten us. Some say that it is a Bioweapon made in a Lab and spread to the world to limit the population (especially the older adults) and bring on purpose an economic crash and a world financial crisis. Whatever it is, Covid-19 is scary and killed so many people already. But what about Coronavirus treatment? The vaccine for Covid-19 in my opinion has failed and it has only succeeded in dividing society. I think the solution is always in nature and more specifically in the bark of a South American tree. Yes, believe it or not, coronavirus can be treated by simple means. At least, people will no longer die.

Covid-19 Natural Treatment:

It was October 11, 2021, and I worked as a bartender in a hotel in Greece. I started having my first symptoms of coronavirus. Weakness, low-grade fever, and sore throat. Two days later, I made a covid test and came positive. Long story short, I had the Delta variant, but I had mild symptoms and correct treatments. I will tell you exactly what I did to treat it and also other things that I discovered during the process. I treated my covid symptoms with rest, not a sexual activity for ten days, vegetable soups, fasting, Vitamin D, oregano oil, and a Mucus & Phlegm Plus Cough Syrup which I made with honey and carrot. I took a drop of the oregano oil in a glass of water three times per day, for cleaning my lungs and a tbsp of the syrup that I made, three times per day to fight phlegm. But here are some other things that I discovered.

Cinchona officinalis Dried Bark:

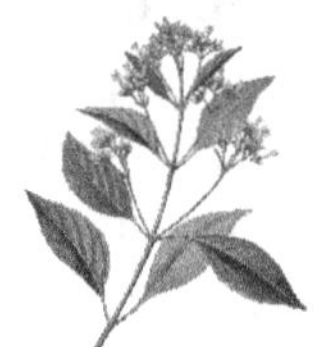

For sure a good diet high in antioxidants, vitamins, minerals, and essential fluids are very important. Vitamin C, Vitamin D, and exercise are some of the best ways to boost the immune system and help with viruses, but what about something more promising? Quinine comes from the bark of the Cinchona tree "native to South America". Two French chemists in 1820, isolated quinine from the cinchona bark and quinine became the best treatment for malaria. The miraculous quinine is the medicine that saved millions of people from malaria. The name quinine comes from the Native American word "Quina" (meaning "sacred bark").

The medicinal properties of the bark of Cinchona have been known for centuries to the Quechua Indians of Peru and Bolivia who ground the bark and drank the water-soluble brine to cure malaria. Chloroquine phosphate (φωσφορική χλωροκίνη), the famous antiviral medication that we use to prevent and treat malaria was discovered by German scientists of Bayer as a substitute (Resochin) synthesis for quinine in 1934. So, the two-quinine advanced synthetic forms are chloroquine and hydroxychloroquine. Hydroxychloroquine is a less toxic derivative of chloroquine. According to some, early results and a clinical study in China, published in the journal Bioscience Trends, Chloroquine phosphate, reduced the duration of infection, improved pulmonary function, and improved pneumonia symptoms compared to the placebo medicine in a sample of 100 patients. It is also important, that chloroquine is a cheap drug and readily available in all countries of the world. Sanofi Pharmaceuticals it is offering to the French government millions of Plaquenil (chloroquine) doses as clinical trials deemed 'promising'. The First Tests are Positive: Patients received a small dose of Chloricin, 600 milligrams daily for six days. ***The results were very encouraging***. "We had the results in the first six days, the measurements showed that patients were negative on the virus tests. Patients were also no longer contagious". I definitely recommend Cinchona officinalis Bark (quinine) instead of chloroquine or hydroxychloroquine. As Cinchona officinalis Bark will have fewer side effects, is less toxic, and is not the synthetic form of the medicine.

Hot and Cold Therapy:

As I'm a big fan of the sauna, I know firsthand the benefits of Hot and Cold Therapy. But I wanted to research more about how hot and cold can affect our health, even if it's by Weather, or topical with cold and hot balms, plasters, oils, creams, or even with other ways like contrast baths and so on. Sometimes we can use hot or cold treatment for different conditions and injuries, and sometimes we can even include both.

Hot and Cold Therapy Types:

Cold and Hot Weather:

Cold and hot weather can affect our health in many ways. Climate and temperature can have huge effects on our bodies. I like to live in warm temperatures more than cold, but I know many people who are the exact opposite. So, let's start with the hot weather first.

Hot Weather Pros:

Living in warm weather has a lot of pluses, but remember moderation is the key. We all know that sunlight exposure increases our body's vitamin D levels. Vitamin D keeps our immune system healthy and helps with a lot of diseases. Death rates are higher in cold climates. Lower blood pressure is also decreased in warm weather. Finally, for me, one of the biggest pros of warm weather is the mood. We all have a better mood during the summer. ***Hot Weather Cons:*** Exhaustion, heatstroke, dehydration, muscle weakness, etc.

Cold Weather Pros:

Cold weather can help us burn more calories and increases brown fat cells, boosts energy, is good for our brain, we get better sleep, is very good for our skin and finally, cool weather is better for breathing. ***Cold Weather Cons***: Cold air can cause asthma or bronchitis to flare up, hypothermia, increased heart rate, more colds, flu, etc.

Topical Analgesic Cold and Hot Creams, Gels, Balms:

It is all depending on what is your condition of pain, as different creams have different ingredients and give different results. For example, Menthol will give you a cooling feeling when applied, will numb sore areas, and help with swelling or arthritis pain. Capsaicin (made from hot chili peppers) will give you a tingling, burning feeling, and Camphor will give you both a burning and cooling feeling. Hot creams, in general, promote blood flow and are useful for painful muscles, joints, and nerves. Cold creams are better for acute chronic pain as they reduce inflammation by slowing blood flow.

Cryotherapy and Thermotherapy:

Both Cryotherapy and Thermotherapy are excellent treatments, but let's see the health benefits of both.

Cryotherapy:

It is also known as cold therapy and is when the body is exposed to extremely cold temperatures for several minutes to relieve muscle pain, inflammation, atopic dermatitis, arthritis, nerve irritation, swelling, dementia, and Alzheimer's disease. You can do both localized cryotherapy and whole-body cryotherapy. Cold therapy can also help with weight loss.

For example, studies showed that whole-body cryotherapy can cause brown fat cell activation which unlike regular old white fat cells burn energy and produce heat. Other treatments like CoolSculpting or Fat Freezing Cryo-lipolysis can freeze the fat cells and can permanently destroy the dead fat cells within several weeks.

Thermotherapy:

Also known as Heat therapy and can be used locally or on the whole body. It reduces stress and tension, relieves soreness and the stiffness of the joints, and can help with many diseases like thrombophlebitis, fibromyalgia, myalgia, and even Cancer.

Contrast Hydrotherapy:

Contrast hydrotherapy or Contrast bath therapy is alternating hot and cold water to initiate cure. You can do that even with your shower, but you will get better results from spas and saunas. Contrast hydrotherapy improves the circulation of the blood and helps the lymphatic system to move and detoxified. Studies have shown that contrast hydrotherapy boosts the immune system, increases metabolism, it helps with conditions like constipation, pain from sports or injuries, and fatigue. It also improves obstructive pulmonary diseases like asthma or bronchitis and helps with Parkinson's disease, fibromyalgia, and rheumatoid arthritis.

Healing Crystals and Stone Massage:

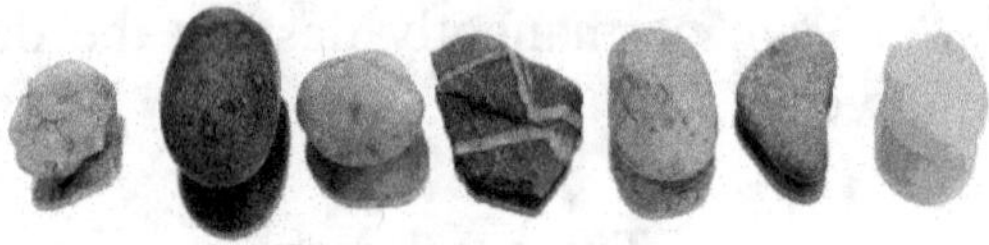

Crystal healing is used as a natural medical technique for many diseases. This therapy is based on two main concepts, the chi or prana, and the chakras. But is crystal healing genuine? Can the crystal stones and gems use for therapeutic purposes? Many people claim that crystal healing is just pseudoscience. Some others state that crystal healing works, but only as a placebo, while others believe that crystal energy is an ancient secret knowledge for healing and power. To be honest, I would never have taken this treatment seriously if I hadn't discovered it by accident in the Ancient Orphic texts. Lithika 'Stones', was written by the ancient Greek Orpheus and it is the first known ancient script dealing with the healing and magical properties of the stones and their ritual practice. A study found that crystals have no healing powers and that is just the placebo effect that works, but believers claim that this study failed, as crystals may take weeks or even months to reach their full healing potential. A crystal does not have any effect on the user until it becomes "one" with a person's energy. Crystals also must discharge and charge before using them again. But, before you think that crystal healing is just a hoax, let me remind you of something very important. Scientific evidence showed that physical metals like gold, silver, platinum, and copper have antibacterial, anti-inflammatory, germicidal, and antimicrobial properties.

Physical metals fight infections, help with wound healing, and so on. So, if metals have all these healing properties, then why do crystal stones and gems that coming also from mother earth don't? Another example is Aura. If you were talking about aura some years ago, they take you for a fool, but today with Kirlian photography we can see that human aura is real. The technique has been known as electrography. Kirlian thought that these images could be used to diagnose illnesses.

Hot Stones and Crystal Massage Treatment:

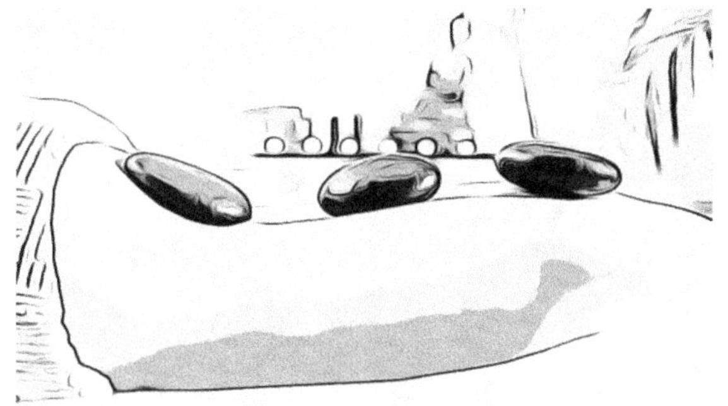

The hot stone massage was practiced in Ancient Greece and Rome. Romans used the stones in Roman baths for healing purposes. The practice of hot stone therapy in Asia started in China 2,000 years ago and came to Southeast Asia much later. During a hot stone massage, volcanic heated stones retain heat and are applied to specific parts of your body for healing and relaxation. Crystal massages assist in rebalancing the patient's chakras and energy field on a vibrational level.

__Hot Stone Health Benefits:__
Relieves muscle pain and improves muscle relaxation. Reduces stress and anxiety. Improves blood circulation. Promotes sleep and increases flexibility.

Enema Colon Cleanse Instructions:

Enemas are very good for a variety of reasons. For me, the most important are detoxification and colon cleanse. One of the reasons that I trust this method, even if the big pharma trying so hard to warn us against it, is because the enema internal cleansing was known from ancient times in Babylonia, Egypt, India, Greece, and China. In Ayurvedic medicine, the enema detox is called Basti. It is a herbal-oil-based enema solution for colon cleanse.

Diet Before Enema:

I recommend doing at least a week of vegan and raw food diet before your enema colon cleanses. Otherwise, performing an enema has no point. I usually follow a lacto-vegetarian diet for four days, including cooked grains, vegetables, and legumes as well as some probiotic foods like kefir, feta, and Greek yogurt, followed by three days of fresh fruit and vegetables. Also, during the past two days, I've sipped on various detox juices containing activated charcoal. For better results do not mix fruits with vegetables in the Juices.

Enema Recipes:

There are many enema recipes, and it all depends on your goals. Lemon juice enema, salt enema, herbs enema, Epsom salt enema, garlic enema, tea enema, milk and molasses enema, olive oil enema, and coffee enema. The coffee recipe, for example, is for liver detoxification rather than colon cleansing. For me, the best enema for colon cleanse is two liters of mildly warm water (37°C) mixed with two teaspoons of sea salt.

Enema Side Effects:

Some enemas, such as coffee and Epsom salt enemas, have more side effects than others. Some evidence suggests that those enemas may be harmful and can cause rectal burns, nausea, infections, vomiting, salmonella, electrolyte imbalance, cramping, proctocolitis, colitis, and even heart failure. Salt-water enema is for sure the safest.

How to do an Enema:

You will need an enema kit and a towel so you can lie down. It is about a 20 to 25 minutes process. It's a good idea to have a free schedule for several hours after the enema because you may need to use the restroom again. It is always better to do an enema after a bowel movement. First, clean your enema kit from any previous use with hot water. Fill your enema bag with about two liters of mildly warm water mixed with two teaspoons of sea salt. To avoid cramps, open the clamp for five seconds to allow the water to purge air from the hose. Hang your enema kit somewhere high enough to allow the water to flow. Lay a towel on the floor and apply some coconut oil to the anus and to the enema nozzle to ease insertion. Finally, lie on the floor on your left side and insert the nozzle of the enema into the rectum.

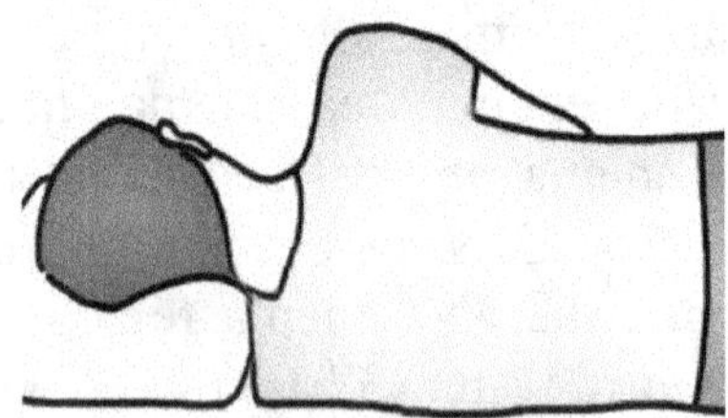

Now release the clamp and allow all the water to enter your rectum. If it's your first time it may feel weird. Try to keep it there for two to five minutes (you may pause and begin again if it is your first time.) Do some massage on your belly to move the water everywhere into your colon. Slowly take out the enema nozzle and go to the bathroom and evacuate. Stay near the toilet for at least 30 minutes to get ready for the next bowel movement. If you feel a little dizzy is completely normal.

What to Eat After an Enema:

Keep it simple, I prefer to eat juicy fruits such as apples to replenish electrolytes and minerals. After 40 minutes, I'll drink kefir to introduce good bacteria into my gut, followed by vegetable soup for lunch. I advise you to do the same.

Gut Detox Benefits:

If you combine a good diet before your enema, you will have more benefits for sure. Here are some gut detox benefits. Improves body well-being, eliminates the toxins from your body, promotes weight loss, boosts energy, increases the body's absorption of nutrients, decreases the risk of colon cancer, protects against constipation, and improves digestion.

Colloidal Silver:

S ome claim that is a risk without benefit, but Silver has been a precious metal for centuries. Since 400 BC Hippocrates describes the antimicrobial properties of silver. This metal has been also used for centuries in Chinese medicine and Ayurveda. It has long been known that the water transferred to silver flakes remains fresh. In the old western days, American cowboys were placing silver dollars in buckets to conserve fresh milk. Another piece of evidence is that a long time ago, families had genuine silver crockeries and silver jugs because they knew that silver has many health benefits. In the 1950s, ionized silver began to be used as a bactericide for water disinfection systems. Dr. Robert Becker demonstrated the antiseptic, antifungal, and disinfecting properties of Colloidal Silver. From the late 1800s to 1938, colloidal silver was prescribed for the treatment of infections. Unfortunately, it lost popularity since the advent of antibiotics.

The Evidence:

Numerous studies reveal the effectiveness of colloidal silver. Here are some examples. Biomedical research has shown that all bacteria, viruses, and fungi can't survive for more than a few minutes with colloidal silver. According to new research, Colloidal Silver operates as a catalyst and neutralizes an enzyme that monocyte bacteria, viruses, and fungi need for oxygen metabolism. Another study at the National Institutes of Health discovered that animals (pigs) treated with Colloidal silver recovered within two days, whereas the skin of the other animals remained inflamed. So yes, Colloidal Silver kills infections and harmful bacteria without destroying the beneficial gut bacteria as antibiotics do.

Is Colloidal Silver Safe to Use?

In October 1996 FDA established that all colloidal silver products are unclassified drugs. In high doses, colloidal silver can cause a rare but not life-threatening condition, called argyria, that turns the skin purple – purple-grey. NCCAM also warns that high consumption of colloidal silver may cause other side effects including headaches, seizures, kidney damage, and stomach distress. Finally, Colloidal silver products may also interact with some medications.

Conclusion: So, is colloidal silver safe to use? A lot of people use colloidal silver annually. If you decide to try colloidal silver, take the safe doses of this product. If you consume the right doses, you will probably not going to turn into a Smurf or have any other side-effect. Colloidal silver is created by tiny silver particles suspended in liquid – usually water. There are various types of products on the market, but be careful most of the companies out there sell ionic silver and not Colloidal Silver. Original Colloidal Silver must be yellow and not colorless like water.

What are the Benefits of Colloidal Silver?

It has antibacterial and antimicrobial properties. Can heal wounds. It's effective for eye/ear or any other infection and has antiviral properties.

Hemorrhoids Treatment:

Hemorrhoids are swollen veins in your lower rectum or anus. Hemorrhoids (αιμορροΐδες) is a Greek word that means veins with blood. Everybody gets Hemorrhoids sometimes and it's nothing to be ashamed of. The FDA estimates that 75% of people will experience hemorrhoids in their life. Now the questions are, what you can do about it? Can Hemorrhoids heal on their own? The short answer is yes.

Hemorrhoids Causes:

•Constipation •Diarrhea •Sitting on the toilet for a long time. •Obesity. •Anal intercourse. •Low-fiber diet. •Pregnancy. •Lifting heavy weights.

Hemorrhoids Symptoms:

•Itching around the anus •Mucus discharge. •Burning, irritation, and pain around the anus. •A sensation that the bowel is not really empty. •Bleeding. •Painful bowel movements.

Can Hemorrhoids Heal on their Own?

For me, this is the best treatment. I mean, every time I had Hemorrhoids, I waited for my Hemorrhoids to heal on their own. If your hemorrhoids are not big, they can clear up on their own in a few days without any treatment, and it doesn't matter if they are internal or external hemorrhoids.

How Long Do Hemorrhoids Last?

Now, the exact duration of the Hemorrhoid healing process depends on several factors, but normally, they may heal within one to two weeks.

How to Help Hemorrhoids to Heal on their Own:
To make the time of the healing process faster, follow these simple Hemorrhoid guidelines. With these guidelines, you have more chances. Eat high-fiber foods, avoid sitting on hard surfaces, washing after using the bathroom. Drink plenty of water. Limit alcohol and spicy foods. Apply aloe vera gel and St. John's wort oil on your Hemorrhoids and leave it for half an hour to absorb, three times a day, until the problem is eliminated. Prevent constipation. Avoid straining during a bowel movement. Use Hemorrhoid ice packs or cold compress as Hemorrhoid cold therapy. Stop lifting weights for a week.

Drumming Health Benefits:

When I was a kid, I loved rock music (I still do) and, I was a drummer in a band. We played for fun and because we were fans of rock music. Today the therapeutic effects of drumming are finally known.

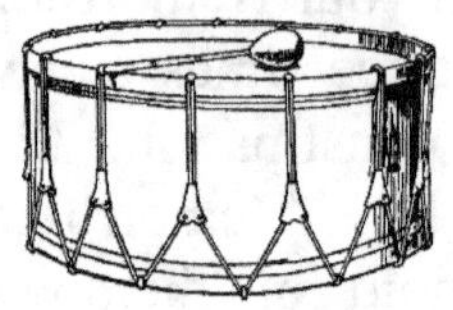

Is Drumming Health Benefits a Real Thing?

Researchers at the Stockholm Institute, who studied the functioning of the drummer's brain, showed that drummers are not only the smartest in a band but smarter than the average person because their brains coordinate four movements per second! Other researchers have found that Drummers have higher levels of a brain substance in the spinal cord and that can help them solve their problems faster and more easily. After some selected questions, it appeared that drummers have a fairly high IQ, and their body produces more white blood cells that protect them from cancer cells. A new study from the Royal College of Music confirms that playing drums and listening to music improves mental health. Drumming can reduce depression by 38%, anxiety by 20%, and improve mental well-being by 16%. This is why music therapy has been invented, which raises the mood and face various mental problems. All musical instruments have enormous benefits for the musicians and their audience, but the drummers, however, pride themselves on being the only ones to coordinate the four extremes at different frequencies.

Drumming Health Benefits:

Playing Drums makes you happy, reduces stress, and helps with the control of chronic pains. Playing Drums boosts the immune system and offers hemispheric coordination. Drumming produces deeper self-awareness by inducing synchronous brain activity. Playing Drums promotes alpha waves and releases negative feelings and emotional trauma. Drumming is a way of meditation and mindfulness. Playing Drums is also a good form of cardio.

Activated Charcoal Detox:

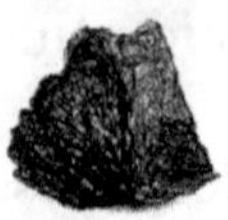

Activated charcoal it's not the same stuff that you use in your barbecue. Activated carbon has oxygen added to it to increase its porosity. We see for the first time the use of charcoal for medicinal purposes in Egypt around 1500 BC but later was used as a water purifier in Chinese, Ayurvedic, and Japanese Medicine. What are the facts and myths about activated charcoal detox? Can activated charcoal detoxify our body? Many websites explain the health benefits of activated charcoal supplements, and we all want to get rid of toxins, but is activated charcoal effective?

Can Activated Charcoal Cleanse
Our Bodies from Alcohol?

Although many doctors use activated charcoal in emergency rooms to treat people who have been poisoned, there is no clear benefit to its everyday use. I saw in a British documentary that some people claimed that AC can help you detox from alcohol. The truth is that only certain substances may adhere to activated charcoal, and alcohol is not one of them. But here is what they don't want you to know. Activated charcoal may not absorb alcohol, but it does help to quickly remove other toxins inside alcohol. As we all know today alcohol includes artificial sweeteners and chemicals and it never comes in a pure form. Another benefit of AC is that according to a study by NCBI for Gastroenterology it alleviates gas & bloating.

Activated Charcoal Detoxification:

There is some evidence that drinking AC can remove chlorine and chlorinated by-products from the water. Now the problem is that some "experts" agree that Detox is pure marketing. But how do we know that these so-called experts are not puppets of the pharmaceutical industry? Another proof of the detoxification benefits of activated charcoal was conducted by the professors (David O. Cooney and Thomas T. Struhsaker). The two professors observed that monkeys on the African island of Zanzibar ate charcoal from burned tree stumps to detoxify. Another obvious benefit of activated charcoal is that it can help people who have been exposed to mold. Mold can cause many diseases like liver and kidney disease, heart disease, depression, headaches, severe respiratory distress, and so on. Finally, if Activated Charcoal can't detoxify, why do they use Carbon filtering throughout the world (Especially in Japan, as Charcoal filter hydration is an old Japanese Tradition) to remove contaminants and impurities? Pesticides, solvents, fluoride, industrial waste, and many other chemicals.

Stop Sinus Drainage and Post Nasal Drip Naturally

Infections with viruses, bacteria, or allergies are the main causes of sinusitis. Common cold and sinusitis have similar signs and symptoms: Cough, sore throat, runny or stuffy nose, nausea, fatigue, pain in the forehead or between the eyes, headache, congestion, and sneezing. Sometimes is so difficult to stop sinus drainage and postnasal drip, (postnasal drip is excess mucus that runs down the back of your nose and into your throat) that's why I will show you some genuinely good natural remedies. Follow these steps one by one if you want to stop your sinus drainage and postnasal drip.

Hot Soup:

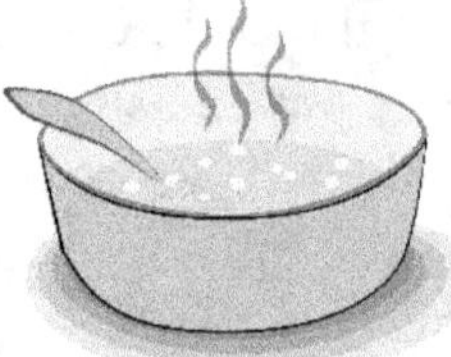

Traditional hot soup is known to cure a common cold. But a hot spicy soup will help you dilute your mucus.

Neti Pot:

It is used in Ayurveda as part of basic daily hygiene which is a therapy that uses a salt and water solution to flush out the nasal passages. A Neti pot with saline water can help thin out mucus and heal yourself.

Camphor Menthol Balm:

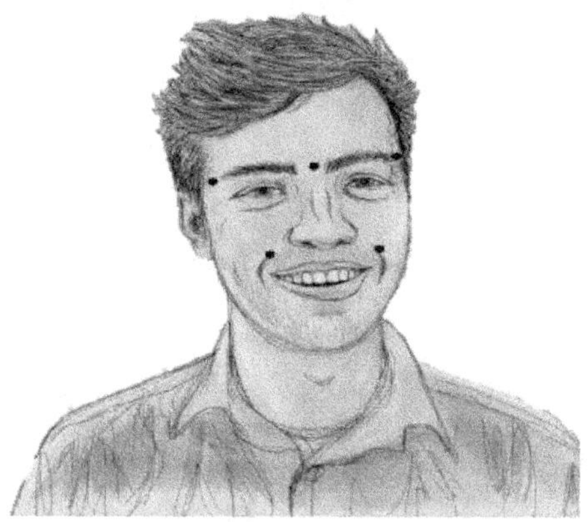

Take a tiger-like balm or cream, add a little to your fingers, and put it to the points we show you in the pictures. This balm will help you to clear mucus.

Sinus Acupuncture:

Press with your fingers the points near your nose and cheekbones. Look at the black spots in the pictures that we made for you and follow the steps. Press these points slowly and gradually. Give some time and take deep breaths slowly in and out. This practice will open your nostrils, and you will breathe easier.

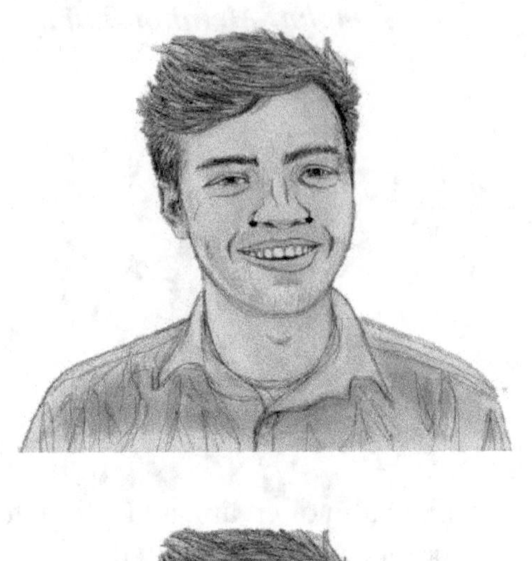

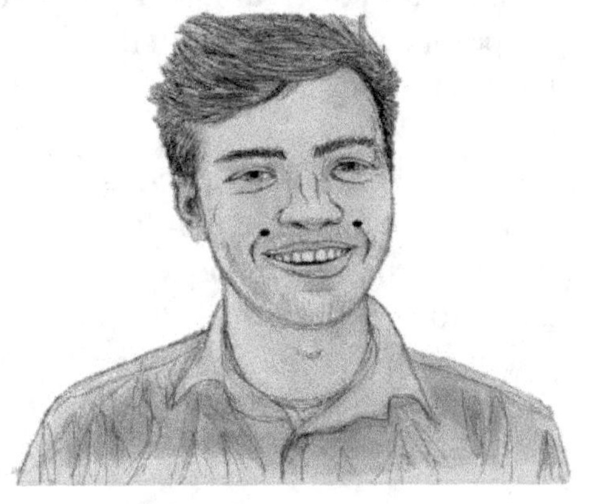

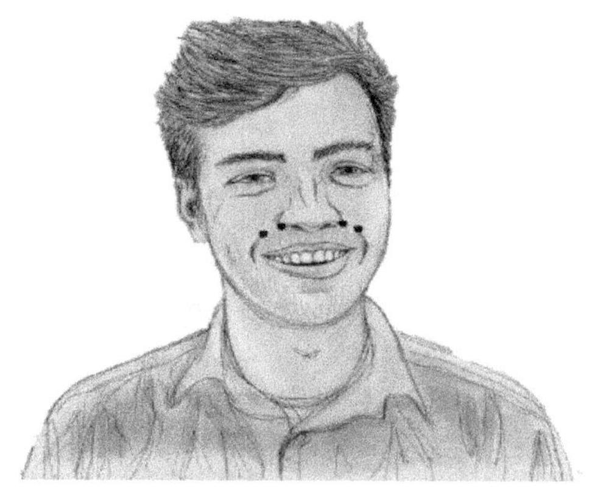

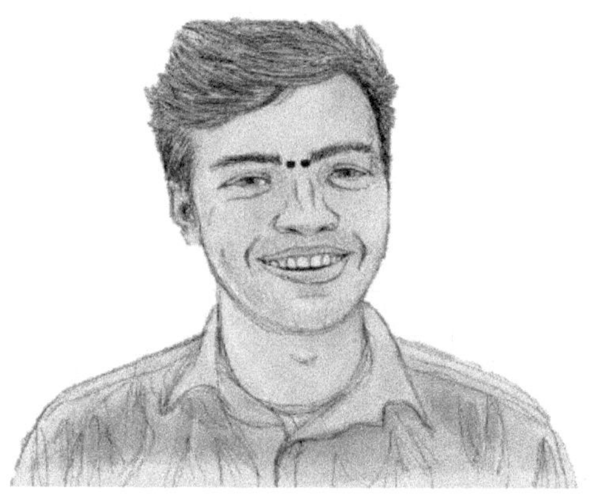

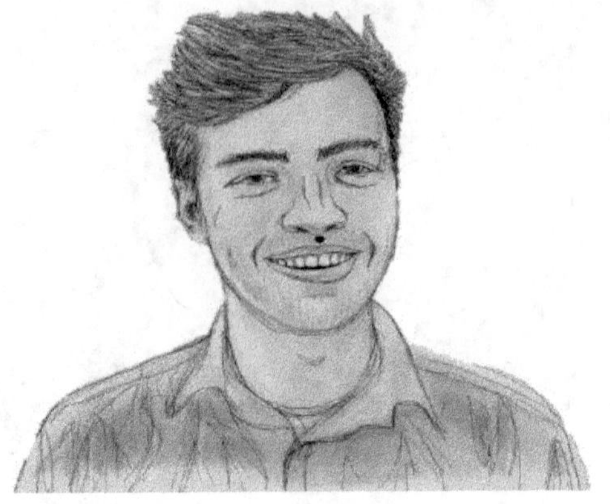

Cure Chronic Nosebleeds with Natural Remedies:

My nosebleeds started when I recovered from Covid. I don't know if it was the rapid test that my pharmacist did or because I blew my nose so hard. But from that day, I had frequent nosebleeds. I tried many natural treatments and some of them really worked. Most nosebleeds (Epistaxis) are not serious. However, frequent or severe nosebleeds can exacerbate conditions, such as anemia. Epistaxis can be classified as anterior or posterior, depending on where it originates.

Anterior Epistaxis:

A nosebleed that starts in the anterior (frontal) area of the nose is referred to as anterior epistaxis. It normally does not cause major harm and is the most typical type of nosebleed.

Posterior Epistaxis:

Bleeding from the superior or posterior nasal cavities is referred to as posterior epistaxis. Although posterior nosebleeds are less frequent than anterior ones, they can be very serious and result in significant blood loss.

How to Stop Nosebleeds:

Even if only one side of your nose is bleeding, clamp both nostrils shut with your thumb and index finger. Use your mouth to breathe and keep pinching for a further five to ten minutes. This technique applies pressure to the nasal septum's bleeding point and frequently stops the flow of blood.

Simply Rules to Prevent Nosebleeds:

Use a humidifier, don't pick your nose, don't drink alcohol, don't smoke, don't lift heavy weights, avoid allergy triggers if you have allergies.

3 Natural Ways to Cure Nosebleeds:

Salty Water:

Today, the saline nasal spray is gaining popularity as a remedy for allergies and sinus issues, but what about nosebleeds? According to a recent study, saltwater is just as effective as the top drug therapies in the world at treating chronic nosebleeds. People with frequent nosebleeds did find relief from commercial nasal sprays and plain saline water.

Maintain Moisture Inside your Nose:

Dryness can cause nosebleeds. Use cotton with pure aloe vera jelly and keep it for ten minutes in your nostrils three times a day.

Nasal Cautery:

In this operation, a medical expert burns or cauterizes a section of the nasal lining to stop the flow of blood. This treatment is the most effective. I did this operation without Nose Anesthesia, as I don't like chemicals in my body, but your doctor will ask you if you want to be numb during this surgery. To seal the leaky blood vessel, your doctor will either use a heated electronic tool (electrocautery) or a substance called silver nitrate. You may have itchiness and soreness in your nose for three to five hours following the surgery.

How to Get Rid of the Flu Naturally:

I'm working in a tourist city and I meet people from many different countries. Unfortunately, some of those carry diseases from other environments. I'm extremely cautious, but it's not always enough. So, if you get sick, the point is to eliminate flu symptoms without poisoning the body with chemicals from drugs While people are contagious to the flu from the first days, the flu symptoms appear later. What is amazing, is that you can get infected by the flu without even knowing it. Flu symptoms include fever, headache, chills and sweats, cough, fatigue, nasal congestion, sore throat, and muscle soreness. So how to make the flu go away faster? What are the best ways to get rid of the flu naturally?

Use Oregano Oil:

Oregano Oil has been used since ancient times. Many scientific studies have found oregano oil to be effective at treating various conditions. Drinking a few drops of oil in juice or water can help you a lot with flu symptoms.

Take Vitamin C:

Vitamin C supplements may boost your immune system to help you fight off your cold and flu symptoms. I prefer food-sourced vitamin C.

Cut out the Sugar:

Sugar suppresses your immune system, so is better to eliminate refined sugar suppresses until the flu is gone.

Vitamin D3:

Get Vitamin D. Get 30 minutes of sunlight on as much bare skin as possible.

Eat Hot Soup:

Vegetable soup is one of the most famous remedies to cure the flu. A soup with good vegetables boosts the immune system.

Garlic and Ginger:

Garlic is a natural antibiotic and helps to kill germs. Ginger has amazing healing properties, and it helps to relieve pain.

Gargle Salt Water:

Salt in warm water can be helpful and can help you to get rid of the flu faster.

Tooth Infection Natural Remedies:

Two months ago, I went to the dentist because I was experiencing severe pain in my upper left jaw. I was having gum problems, so I asked the doctor if my pain was coming from a tooth or my gums. The doctor determined that my pain was caused by my gums after a thorough examination. So, I went home and started treating my gums like always with natural remedies.

Tooth Infection Natural Remedies:

I began eating a lot of green raw vegetables and fruits, and I applied a little garlic and clove oil to my gums to relieve the pain. I did some oil pulling and brushed my teeth with mastic gum toothpaste. Finally, I cleaned my mouth with warm salt water mixed with baking soda and so on. After two days, the infection healed with all these natural remedies. But unfortunately, three weeks later, I drank alcohol, and the problem returned. Long story short, the infection was not from my gums, I went to another doctor, who told me that my infection was caused by a tooth. I had tooth canal pain. My first dentist misdiagnosed me.

Symptoms of Tooth Abscess:

Pain when chewing, mild fever, teeth may get sensitive to hot or cold, swelling of the gum over the infected tooth, swollen glands of the neck, and swollen area of the upper or lower jaw. ***Conclusions***: If your tooth infection is at the start, then try to avoid antibiotics, as antibiotic therapy can kill the good bacteria as well. Antibiotics can also promote a new infection with unwanted bacteria colonizing somewhere else in the body. If the infection is really bad then take at least Amoxicillin. Amoxicillin is the only semi-synthetic (half-natural) antibiotic.

TOOTH EXTRACTION HEALING:

So here I am, finally at the dentist's office, to have this tooth extracted. I am always nervous before dentists. Fortunately, this doctor was very professional and the whole progress was not painful at all. When we were finished, the doctor gave me some recommendations. So, I thought it would be a good idea to share these tips with everyone.

1. Bite friendly on the gauze doctor gave you to help stop the bleeding for at least 2 hours.
2. If you have difficulty feeling your lips or tongue due it to numbness, don't worry as it will be a temporary feeling.
3. Do not suck on the straw and avoid rinsing or spitting during the first 24 hours.
4. Do not brush your teeth the day that you did the surgery.
5. If possible, chew on the opposite side of your extraction site.
6. Do not drink alcohol for 24 hours.
7. If you smoke, do not smoke at least for a day.
8. If you have facial swelling after the surgery place ice packs on the swelling site.
9. Try not to exercise for 24 hours after your tooth has been extracted.

Why you should not Spit After Tooth Extraction?

The doctor told me that is better to not spit after the tooth extraction and that is recommended to swallow the blood. It helps our body to understand that we bleeding and as a result, our body will heal faster.

Periodontal Gum Disease:

Periodontal disease is a bacterial infection of the gums and is caused by bacteria and other particles. Many of us have it without even noticing it. These bacteria create sticky plaque on the teeth. Untreated gingivitis (inflammation of the gums), can cause periodontitis that eventually leads to other medical conditions and even tooth loss. This infection damages the soft tissue and destroys the bone that supports our teeth.

Periodontal Gum Disease Natural Treatments:

Sea Salt:
Dissolve a small amount of sea salt in a cup of warm water.

Tea Bags:
Apply tea bags into the gums for 5 minutes.

Garlic:
Apply garlic on your gums for 2 minutes every day.

Oil Pulling:
Try Oil Pulling for 5 minutes every day.

Vitamins:
Flavonoids, zinc, and vitamins E, C, and D can help a lot.

Baking Soda:
Brush your teeth with baking soda.

Tobacco:
Tobacco fights the infection.

Best Periodontal Gum Disease Natural Treatment:
This is the best remedy for gum disease. Make this natural toothpaste and clean your teeth five times a week before you sleep. For the other two days, brush your teeth with your everyday toothpaste. In the morning, do oil pulling and clean the oil from your teeth with water mixed with sea salt. For this natural toothpaste, you will need twelve spoons of baking soda, six spoons of sea salt, five spoons of olive oil, two melted garlic cloves, one teaspoon of mint, a half teaspoon of turmeric, and half lemon. Mix and melt the ingredients together and put them in a small bowl. Turmeric and garlic may help you treat a recurring gum disease due to their strong anti-inflammatory properties. The sea salt, the olive oil, and the lemon kill the bad bacteria, and the baking soda whitens the teeth.

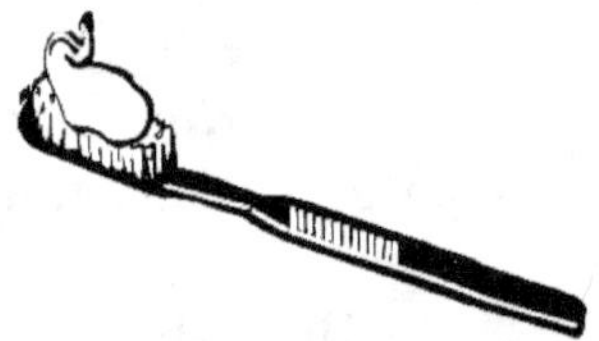

How to Make a Natural Homemade Toothpaste:
That is another easy way to make toothpaste. Just mix equal amounts of coconut oil, salt, your favorite essential oil (peppermint is a good idea), and baking soda. Research said that toothpaste containing sodium bicarbonate has a better plaque removal effect than toothpaste without it. Baking soda is 100% sodium bicarbonate. Technically, Sodium Bicarbonate is a natural by-product. This recipe allows you to leave out all the harmful ingredients that toothpaste is made of. Fluoride, for example, is considered toxic when ingested at high levels. Even the "natural" toothpaste that is sold at the organic-bio stores is not natural.

Common Toothpaste Chemicals:

Fluoride, Triclosan, Sodium Lauryl Sulfate, Propylene Glycol, DEA.

Alternative Recipe Ingredients:

2/3 cup baking soda. 1 tsp fine sea salt. 2 drops of your favorite essential oil (peppermint or orange is a good idea). 10 tsp of coconut oil.

How to Make the Homemade Toothpaste:

Mix three parts baking soda with one part table salt, add 10 tsp of coconut oil, and a few drops of your favorite essential oil. Store this natural toothpaste in a covered container.

Alcohol as Medicine and as Asthma Treatment:

A century ago, alcohol was legitimate medicine. Moderate drinking can offer some health benefits, but if you like drinking, keep it moderate. Alcohol is used in medicine as an antidote, antiseptic, and disinfectant.

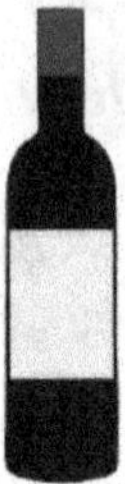

Many naturopathic doctors use alcohol externally to cure common colds and muscle pains. Studies have consistently shown that people who don't consume any alcohol at all tend to die before people who do. But if you don't like alcohol, don't start drinking for the possible health benefits. Usually people drink to socialize, celebrate, and relax. Like most things in life, you must have control of alcohol. While a small amount of alcohol may provide health benefits, drinking excessively can cause major health problems.

Alcohol Abuse can Cause:
•Dizziness •Slow speech •Loss of coordination skills •Confusion •Inability to judge clearly •Poor vision •Blackouts •Depression •Violence •Vomiting •Irregular heartbeat.

Health Problems of Long-Term Alcohol Abuse:
•Anemia •Liver damage •Brain damage •Depression •Increased risk of suicide •High blood pressure •Increased risk of stroke •Increased risk of cardiovascular disease •Stomach ulcers •Blood vessel disorders •Cancer •Gout.

Is Alcohol Natural or Synthetic?
Alcohol is a natural substance. Ethanol is produced naturally by yeasts from sugars through a process called fermentation. Even for people with GERD and Gastritis alcohol has some benefits. A study reported that moderate alcohol doesn't seem to be a risk factor for GERD. For me moderate alcohol consumption has some benefits.

Alcohol Benefits:
•It can lower your risk of cardiovascular disease.
•Alcohol reduces the risk of Diabetes.
•It helps with common cold.
•Small amounts of alcohol can improve libido.
•It helps with Gallstones.
•It decreases the chances of developing Dementia.
•It helps with a sore throat.

Alcohol as Asthma Treatment:

Before I started treating myself with natural remedies, I had asthma, GERD, allergies, and chronic rhinosinusitis. Alcoholic drinks used since ancient times for asthma treatment and other respiratory conditions. I also noticed that moderate alcohol helped me with my asthma and allergies as it clears the chest and throat mucus. Consumption of alcoholic drinks is likely to encourage or suppress the symptoms of asthma in some individuals. In my opinion, that depends on how much you drink, moderate or heavy. According to Danish researchers at Bispebjerg Hospital in Copenhagen, drinking alcohol can reduce the risk of allergies and asthma. Also, the highest risk of asthma was observed in people who drank rarely or never. Heavy drinkers also had an increased risk of asthma development.

Other modern research, point out that alcohol may afford relief in asthma and that may be used in the future to treat patients who do not respond to conventional drugs. Several studies have shown that moderate doses of alcohol can help to dilate the airways that become restricted during an asthma attack.

Conclusion:

Moderate doses of alcohol can help with respiratory diseases. Moderate Alcohol can help to relieve stress and is good for blood circulation. We all know the connection between stress and asthma. Don't forget that studies have shown that more than 75 percent of adults with asthma also have GERD. Heavy drinking will make you sick in the end. Everyone has their limits and moderation is the key.

Beer Therapy and H Pylori:

Can Beer Fights Inflammation?

As reported in a study published in Molecular Nutrition and Food Research in 2009, bitter acids in beer are powerful inflammation fighters and may improve digestion. According to another study, (Liam J. Murray, MD, Queens University of Belfast, U.K.), wine and beer are rich in compounds with antibacterial activity! People who drink moderate wine and beer (a few weekly glasses) may help themselves get rid of the bacteria H. pylori. Murray's team found out that you need at least three to four glasses of wine per week to get protection from the H. pylori bacteria. Unfortunately, those who preferred hard liquor were out of luck to protect themselves from the bug.

Murray conclusion:

Wine and beer increase the secretion of stomach acids and activate the enzyme pepsin, which then aids indigestion. Finally, a 2012 study published in the Journal of Agricultural and food chemistry found also that beer triggered the release of gastric acid from stomach cells. As I mentioned before, Gastric acid is the key to controlling the growth of dangerous gut bacteria. That explains a lot to me, as sometimes I feel better the next day after a couple of beers.

Beer Therapy: Which Beers are the Best for your Health?

Beers that are under the German law called "Reinheitsgebot" are a good choice. This law requires all beers to be only produced with a core ingredient list of water, hops, malted barley, yeast, or wheat. Another choice is the Certified Organic Beers, which includes a law to not contain GMOs and other harmful additives.

Rhinitis Natural Treatments:

I tried for a long time now to solve the mysterious link between allergies, LPR, asthma, and sinusitis… I went for an inhalant allergy test and found that I have an allergy to dust mites and cockroaches. But if I'm allergic to dust mites and cockroaches, then why when the weather changes, I feel in a bad mood and why do I have difficulty breathing every time I smell chemical odors? Is it possible to have allergic rhinitis and non-allergic rhinitis at the same time? The answer is YES! You can have both, and it is called mixed rhinitis! Non-allergic rhinitis can co-exist with allergic rhinitis and is referred to as mixed rhinitis. 80% of people with rhinitis have "mixed" allergic and non-allergic rhinitis. The problem is that there is not any info on the internet about mixed rhinitis or how to treat it.

Mixed Rhinitis Natural Treatments:

Antihistamine and intranasal topical corticosteroids can relieve the symptoms in both, allergic and non-allergic rhinitis, but long-term use of intranasal topical corticosteroids can cause side effects, such as hypertension, ulcers in the nasal mucosa, cataract, glaucoma, weight gain, osteoporosis, hyperlipidemia, headache, and insomnia. So, what are the best alternative treatments for mixed rhinitis?

Know your Triggers and Avoid your Allergen:

Reduce allergens such as dust mites, cockroaches, mold, pollen, pet hair, fur, or feathers. In some people, eating spicy food, exercise, air pollutants, exposure to cold or dry air, or strong smells can trigger rhinitis.

Bromelain Pineapple:

Studies have found that bromelain helps reduce nasal swelling and thinning mucus. Bromelain is an enzyme derived from the stems of pineapples, it exists in all fresh plants and fruits, but pineapple is the best way to consume natural sources of bromelain.

Flavonoids and Quercetin:

Flavonoids are good for allergies. Quercetin is a flavonoid widely distributed in nature. Studies show that Quercetin helps to block the release of histamine that causes inflammation.

Mangosteen:

Mangosteens have xanthones that eliminate the histamine reactions in the body.

Rinse your Nasal Passages and Blow your Nose Regularly:

Neti pots are designed for flushing out the sinuses. Use one or just clean your nose every morning with boiled water and salt.

Vitamin C:

Vitamin C boosts our immune system and has antihistamine properties.

Tonsillitis Natural Treatments:

Tonsillitis can be caused by a viral or bacterial infection. In rare cases, tonsillitis can also be caused by the Epstein-Barr virus, which causes glandular fever. A sore throat is the most common of all tonsillitis symptoms. Other symptoms are cough, fatigue, fever, and painful swallowing. Tonsillitis is contagious and may spread by physical contact or droplets in the air.

Infectious Mononucleosis – Glandular Fever:

Infectious Mononucleosis is normally caused by Epstein–Barr virus. It is known as the kissing disease from its transmission by saliva. The characteristic symptoms of infection with EBV include fever, headache, fatigue, malaise, muscle weakness, and sore throat.

Chamomile, Garlic, Salt, and Balsamic Vinegar:

I know this 4-ingredient recipe works because I cured my ex-girlfriend a few years ago. Make chamomile tea and pour it into a bottle. Add three cloves of garlic, a tablespoon of salt, and three drops of balsamic vinegar. Stir the mixture for an hour and gargle at least four times a day to clear your throat and fight the infection!

Propolis:

Another good remedy for Tonsillitis or Infectious Mononucleosis is propolis. Propolis is quite effective when sprayed right into the throat and combats infection.

Get rest:
Get lots of rest at home.

Fluids:
Drink liquids and eat soups. Mix vegetables or fruits and
make fresh juices.

UTI Natural Treatments:

Swimming pools are full of bacteria like E. coli that are caused by children's and adults' urine. Almost all swimming pools contain a high concentration of chlorine to keep the water free of contagious bacteria. A study published in 2016 showed that to some sensitive people these chemicals can be quite irritating and can cause chemical urethritis, which usually resolves on its own in just a day or two without treatment. Unfortunately, these chemicals sometimes are not enough to keep the swimming pools clean, and you can get a urinary tract infection from swimming in a public pool! UTI typically starts in the urethra but can also be an infection in any part of your urinary system. Women are at greater risk of developing a UTI than men. About half of all women will experience a UTI at some point in their lifetime.

Symptoms:

A need to urinate more often. A burning sensation when urinating. Cloudy urine. Passing frequent, small amounts of urine. Urine that smells. Back pain. Nausea.

UTI Natural Treatments:

Drink plenty of water and consume a spoonful of Reiki Honey three times per day. Empty your bladder. Drink pineapple (bromelain) shakes and eat probiotic foods. Get vitamin C from fruits like the Indian Gooseberry (Amla). Drink a glass of water with a teaspoon of Baking Soda.

Best Alternatives to Botox:

Botox is made from the bacteria that cause botulism. Botulism is a rare but serious paralytic illness. In smaller doses, this neurotoxin can treat a lot of medical disorders and temporarily reduces muscle activity. In large doses, Botox will cause botulism.

Is Botox Natural?

Botox is a natural treatment coming from bacteria, and since bacteria are natural, Botox is considered a natural treatment.

Why do I Need Alternatives if Botox is Natural?

Botox isn't something to take lightly. Unfortunately, some people have adverse reactions to Botox injections. Side effects of Botox include diarrhea, allergic reactions, itching, difficulty swallowing, headache, neck or back pain, muscle stiffness, shortness of breath, nausea, weakness, stomach pain, loss of appetite, muscle weakness, pain, bruising, bleeding, redness, or swelling, fever and cough. At the same time, Mother Nature provides a lot of other inexpensive, without side effects alternatives.

Bee Venom:

Bee venom has been used by many well-known celebrities, like Kate Middleton. Bee venom is medicinal and used to treat rheumatoid arthritis, multiple sclerosis, nerve pain, tendonitis, and so on.

Aloe Vera:

Aloe contains a lot of amino acids minerals and vitamins. It is not a secret that the gel of Aloe Vera leaf can increase the body's natural collagen production. Clean your face first and just apply Aloe Vera gel directly to your skin and use it as a mask for 15 minutes.

Egg Whites:

To begin, separate the egg white from the yolk. The egg white should be beaten till firm and look white and foamy. Use warm water to wash your face. Apply the mask to your face and leave it there for 15 minutes. Finally, use warm water to rinse the skin.

Cornstarch, Carrot Juice, and Sour Cream Mix:

Dissolve the cornstarch and pour it into a cooking pot. Then add 100 ml of water inside. Cook until you get a thick mixture. Cool the mixture and add the sour cream and the fresh carrot juice. Wash your face and apply the Botox cream to your face. Leave it on for 20 minutes.

100% Soft-prepared Chalk Herbal Powder:

One of the best natural Botox alternatives that I have tried is the Soft-prepared chalk powder Scrub Mask. Unfortunately, you can't find it easily. Thais have been using soft-prepared chalk for many decades to attain smooth skin.

Natural Remedies for Gastritis:

I suffered from chronic gastritis for many years. Gastritis can either be mild or acute. Gastritis is characterized by pre-ulcerative inflammation of the lining of the stomach and atrophying of the mucosal membranes. Many people feel upper abdominal discomfort, and others may not experience symptoms at all. Gastritis inflammation may be caused by trauma, poor nutrition, drugs, (especially aspirin), immune system disorders, and viral or bacterial infections. I tried so hard to avoid western medicine drugs and I followed some Ayurvedic and Unani medicine remedies that indeed helped me. Therefore, these are the treatments I have so far found to be effective.

Lifestyle Changes:
Start a gastritis diet. Eliminate smoking, caffeine, alcohol, soft drinks, and spicy foods.

Kill H Pylori Bacteria:
Make sure you don't have H Pylori bacteria. H. Pylori is a common gastric pathogen that causes gastritis. You can treat H. pylori with manuka honey, broccoli sprouts, and probiotics.

Potato:
A half-cup of potato juice before meals. It is one of the best natural treatments for gastritis.

Rest:
Rest is the best cure for Gastritis.

Licorice and Artichoke Tea:
Licorice has natural antioxidant properties that can help you with gastritis pain. Prepare licorice and artichoke tea to relieve nausea, vomiting, and stomach pain.

Coconut water:
Coconut water has a lot of minerals and it's very beneficial in removing toxic radicals from the body.

Tamarind:
Is one of the most highly prized natural foods in South Asia. Tamarind is used as a laxative and to alleviate stomach discomfort.

Fennel.
Drink fennel juice or chew roasted fennel after meals to relieve gastritis.

Chamomile:
Chamomile tea is one of the most effective herbal medicines in treating gastritis.

Vitamin B-12:
Vitamin B-12 is the largest and most complex vitamin currently known to humans

Probiotics:
Probiotics act as both preventive and curative aids for gastritis.

Chios Mastic Gum:
Chios mastic is used, for stomach and intestinal ulcers and is one of the best natural treatments for H-Pylori.

Aloe Vera:
Aloe vera has anti-inflammatory properties. Recent research showed that purified aloe vera juice is an effective treatment for reducing gastritis symptoms.

Is Turmeric Good for Acid Reflux and Gastritis?

Turmeric is the spice that gives curry its yellow color and makes the American mustard yellow. Today science started to back up what countries such as India and Sri Lanka have long known, that this spice is a medicine. Turmeric is a herb that belongs to the ginger family and a spice that is native to Asian countries, especially India. Curcumin is the main substance in turmeric. Turmeric has also a long history of medicinal use in traditional Chinese medicine. It is used, for the treatment of liver disease, joint pains, skin problems, gastrointestinal and respiratory ailments.

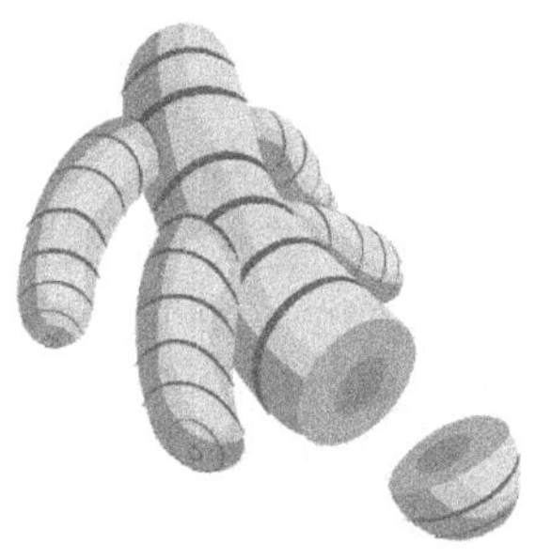

Turmeric and Asthma:

This Root has curcumin, which is an antioxidant that reduces inflammation by lowering the levels of two inflammatory enzymes, called LOX and COX-2.

Turmeric Acid Reflux and Stomach Ulcers:

Many people talk about the benefits and the anti-inflammatory, and antioxidant properties of turmeric and how good it is for our stomach, but as an ex-stomach patient with GERD esophagitis, and gastritis, I can assure you that too much turmeric can be harmful. We have two different opinions about the medicinal properties of turmeric in stomach diseases. Some doctors agree that this root may not help so much with the treatment of acid reflux and stomach ulcers and that in fact, there is some evidence that it may increase stomach acid and make the existing ulcers worse. On the other hand, turmeric can make the gallbladder release necessary enzymes that help us digest our food. Digestive enzymes can help with many abdomen problems like gas, bloating, upset stomach, etc. In my opinion, the truth is somewhere in the middle. Turmeric is good for stomach problems, but too much turmeric can make your GERD or stomach ulcers worse. I went to a naturopathic doctor in Thailand once and asked for a gastritis herbal medicine. He had a turmeric and banana-based herbal supplement for gastritis that worked. When I questioned him about the advantages of bananas, he told me that banana reduces the acidity of turmeric. Perhaps that's one way to benefit from turmeric without the side effects.

Turmeric and Gastritis:
Turmeric contains curcumin, which is a polyphenol with antioxidant, anti-inflammatory, antifungal, and antibacterial properties. As an antioxidant and anti-inflammatory, it can lower the inflammatory enzyme levels in the body and protect us from cell damage caused by free radicals. But not more than 600 mg. Otherwise, you may get acid reflux. Another problem with too much Turmeric is that it may increase the risk of bleeding (no so good for gastritis patients).

Turmeric and Helicobacter Pylori Bacteria:
Turmeric is highly effective at Killing H Pylori. Eradication of H.pylori could help prevent gastritis. Turmeric is somehow good for inflammatory diseases like gastritis, arthritis, fibromyalgia, and so on, but for sure, this root will work better by eating a small amount first. As previously mentioned, turmeric is acidic and is considered a trigger for gastric acid. Many people can experience nausea, stomach upset, and diarrhea. Except for the turmeric-induced gastric issues, gallbladder problems were also reported.

Licorice Root for Stomach Problems:
Licorice is one of my favorite medicinal plants. It has a characteristic sweet taste due to a sweetener called glycyrrhizinic acid. This substance is 50 times sweeter than sugar. Licorice Root contains a lot of healthy compounds like Glycyrrhizic acid, plant sterols, flavonoids, coumarins, volatile oils, glycosides, asparagine, and anethole. I use licorice when my Gastroesophageal Reflux rise. Licorice helps the stomach to create a protective barrier that stops acid to reach the esophagus. This root has an impressive list of well-documented uses and has been used in both Eastern and Western medicine. It is also known as sweet root and Gan Zao

in Chinese. In the 1st century, the physician Dioscorides gave the botanical name γλυκόριζα (sweet root). The Roman Pliny recommended the consumption of licorice to combat hoarseness of the voice and alleviation hunger and thirst. In the 13th century, licorice extract was used as a remedy for sore throats, coughs, and congestion. In the 18th century, Napoleon Bonaparte chewed licorice as a remedy for his stomach problems. Arabs used it as a cough suppressant. Theophrastus, in the 3rd century, found that it is one of the best treatments for asthma and dry cough. Today Licorice root is used for a variety of conditions and it's known for its anti-inflammatory, antibacterial, antispasmodic, and antioxidant activities.

Stomach Ulcers:

Licorice root is suggested as a treatment for stomach ulcers. Studies have shown that Licorice has anti-H. pylori effects.

GERD and Chronic Gastritis:

Licorice root is used, to relieve symptoms of stomach acid and heartburn. This root is very effective in Gastroesophageal reflux and chronic gastritis treatment.

Upper Respiratory Infections:

The use of licorice for sore throat, bronchitis, cough, and respiratory infections is well known. Don't forget that GERD can trigger asthma symptoms as Asthma and acid reflux often occur together.

LPR and Acid Reflux Natural Treatments:
Most of the time, acid reflux drugs are made the pepsin reflux worse and not better. Proton pumps can lead to severe infections. Researchers said that some Acid-Reflux drugs may link to Pneumonia. Some of them are Nexium, Prilosec, and Prevacid. Here are some acid reflux natural cures without side effects.

Lifestyle Changes:
Start an acid reflux diet and lose weight, relax, and eat your food slowly, don't lie down after eating, quit smoking and stop soft drinks, limit alcohol, caffeine, and spicy foods. Finally, elevate your bed at least 6-8 inches (15-20 centimeters), or sleep with an extra pillow (not recommended if you have neck problems). Those are some of the most effective lifestyle treatments for GERD.

Kill H Pylori Bacteria:
As I said above, make sure you don't have H Pylori bacteria, which can cause acid reflux. Most people don't realize they have H. pylori infection. H. pylori causes several digestive problems, including ulcers. You can treat H. pylori with antibiotics.

Probiotics:
It shouldn't be a surprise that happy bacteria may help with GERD. Probiotics are organisms such as bacteria or yeast that improve health. Researchers show that probiotics speed up gastric emptying, so there is less chance of excess acid production and reflux.

Vitamin D:

Are you getting enough Vitamin D? Vitamin D is one of the best LPR natural treatments. Many people feel better in summer than in winter. Vitamin D is a hormone rather than a vitamin and is made by our body as we are exposed to sunlight.

Baking Soda:

Baking Soda is one of the most popular natural remedies for acid reflux. Sometimes it helps me a lot after a heavy meal, together with walking. Another way that Baking Soda is helpful is when you have heartburn after drinking alcohol.

Chew Mastic Gum After Meals:

It's known that chewing gum stimulates saliva production, which helps to neutralize stomach acid. Gum chewing also encourages frequent swallowing, which clears irritating acid from the esophagus faster. If you have h pylori with your acid reflux as I had, then one of the best chewing gums is Chios mastic gum. Mastic is a 100% natural product.

Exercise:

Hard exercises like running can agitate your digestive tract and provoke reflux. Low-impact exercises such as walking can be beneficial. Wait at least two hours after eating to work out.

Balanitis Natural Remedies:

Balanitis (a Greek word meaning inflammation of the acorn) can be caused by a variety of factors. It is an allergic reaction or skin irritation. It usually happens when the skin of the penis is irritated by the build-up of a cheesy material called smegma. Smegma is a natural lubricant that keeps the penis moist. In short, if your penis is swollen, itchy, and red, you probably have a Balanitis fungal infection (also known as Candida, yeast) or a bacterial infection like streptococcal bacteria. Candidiasis is a fungal infection that can affect the genitals.

Poor Hygiene:

Poor hygiene is one of the most common causes of balanitis. The best treatment methods are to become more hygienic, lose weight if you are overweight, or manage your diabetes.

Apple Cider Vinegar:

Boost your immune system by eating vinegar mixed with honey and water after a meal.

Chamomile Tea Mixed with Green Tea:

The area under the foreskin (prepuce) needs to be cleaned daily with warm water. Clean it with chamomile tea mixed with green tea, water, and a little vodka. Make a bottle of one liter and used every day.

Coconut Oil:

Coconut oil is very effective at killing candida yeast. It is high in lauric acid and caprylic acid, which makes it an anti-bacterial and anti-fungal.

Manuka Honey:

Manuka honey has well-documented antimicrobial and antifungal properties. (Apply it as a cream).

Garlic:

Garlic contains a compound called ajoene, a powerful antifungal. Crush garlic, mixed with coconut or olive oil and make a poultice to put on the area of infection.

Natural Deodorant Recipe:

The History Of deodorants is long. Many ancient civilizations used different techniques and made deodorizing experiments for thousands of years. Egyptians applied scented oils under the arms to prevent odor. In Asia, they used mineral salts in the armpit to kill bacteria growing and prevent bad smells. Most Natural Medicine Websites will give you some hard recipes with Shea Butter, Arrowroot, and Coconut Oil. My idea is easier. This simple homemade recipe is chemical-free, won't irritate the skin, and kills odor-causing bacteria. PEGs, aluminum, hormone-disrupting fragrance, synthetic ingredients, petrochemicals, and antibacterials are what most famous deodorants contain.

Recipe Ingredients:

One Spoon of Baking Soda.
100 Proof Vodka.
Your Favorite Essential Oils.

Recipe Instructions:

Buy any famous deodorant and use it until finished. Next, open the lid and fill it with the 100-proof vodka, add one spoon of baking soda and in the end, add some of your favorite essential oils. The orange essential oil is recommended. Orange and a little bit of peppermint are what I'm using most of the time. I hope you enjoy this homemade idea.

Aromatherapy Properties and Uses:

Studies have shown that aromatherapy either by inhalation or when used in massage therapy can improve sleep quality and lower blood pressure. Aromatherapy alone will not cure an illness but may help with your symptoms and affect your mood. Aromatherapy can have mood-enhancing effects. The best way to harness the power of aromas is to use organic essential oils. It's hard to know which essential oils are the original and which are not. Holistic aromatherapy does not include the use of synthetic products.

Negatives in Aromatherapy:

Some people think that aromatherapy synthetic oils may do more harm than good. Chia-Nan University of Pharmacy and Science warned that negative effects cannot be neglected. Certain chemicals in the synthetic oils, called volatile organic compounds, mix with the air to form secondary organic aerosols. Organic aerosols can cause eye and airway irritation. The study measured the volumes of certain secondary organic aerosols during massages in two spas in Taiwan.

Pure Essential Oils Properties:
Essential oils have oxygenating properties.
Aroma oils are a natural anti-inflammatory.
Essential oils can support your immune system.
Aromatherapy can protect you from a hostile environment
that has bacteria, fungus, parasites, and so on.
Essential oils are high in antioxidants.
Aromatherapy can have mood-enhancing effects.
Essential oils regenerate skin.

Fatty Liver Disease Natural Treatments:

Most people with Non-alcoholic fatty liver only carry a small amount of fat in their liver. That means that a simple fatty liver can be a completely benign condition that usually does not lead to any liver damage. In many cases is linked to being obese or overweight. Actually (NAFLD) is a condition that causes fat inside the liver cells. Although non-alcoholic fatty liver is very common, it doesn't mean that we must not treat the condition. Doctors use your medical history and a physical exam. Tests include imaging and blood tests, and sometimes even a liver biopsy. Most persons with NAFLD are asymptomatic, but as the disease is linked to being overweight, patients have an increased risk of atherosclerosis and cardiovascular disease. With the right treatments, we can improve steatosis and prevent the development of fibrosis.

Weight Loss:
Gradual weight loss and regular exercise.

Control of Diseases:
Control of diabetes, hypertension, and hyperlipidemia if present.

Avoid Alcohol:
Many experts recommend restricting alcohol, but if you still drinking, take at least two or three alcohol-free days a week.

Stop Eating Sugar:
Eating too much sugar affects your liver.

Grapefruit:
Grapefruit increases the natural cleansing processes of the liver.

Leafy Green Vegetables:
One of the best allies in cleansing the liver.

Lemons-Limes:
Drinking lemons or limes in the morning helps stimulate the liver.

Dandelion:
Dandelion is an extremely powerful liver cleanser.

Milk Thistle:
Actually, it has to be number one on the list. The best non-alcoholic fatty liver natural treatment is milk thistle.

Remove Toxins from Your Body:
Consider flushing toxins from your system with the help of a detox diet.

Vitamins E and C:
Vitamins E and C are both antioxidants that can help you promote your liver health.

Glutathione and N-Acetyl Cysteine – NAC:
As mentioned, NAC (N-acetyl-cysteine) helps our body to produce glutathione. Glutathione is the most important antioxidant in the body. This antioxidant plays a crucial role in detoxification as it gives the ability of our liver to detoxify from harmful chemicals. NAC increases liver blood flow and improves liver function. It can fight free radicals even without glutathione.

How to Unclog a Sink Naturally:

I know it's something common, but a clogged sink can be a real headache. It's usually caused by little hair, dirt, and other nasty stuff. But don't worry, you're not alone and this simple recipe works like a charm! It is always better to use natural methods for cleaning. Just before you begin, make sure to remove any dirt from your Sink. If you want to unclog your sink naturally you will need only three ingredients.

Ingredients:

1 cup of Salt:
1 cup of baking soda:
1 cup of Vinegar:
For better results pour some boiling water at the end.

Instructions:

Remove the drain cover. Pout on the drain the salt and the baking soda. In the end, pour down the vinegar into the drain over the salt and baking soda. The mixture will bubble like a volcano. Pour some boiling water at the end. Wait for two minutes. This is the incredible power of baking soda, vinegar, and salt combined!

Dengue Fever Guidelines:

Knowledge of health, is one of the most serious issues for travelers, especially when you visit a third-world country. You may be familiar with the condition known as dengue fever if you reside in or have traveled to a tropical region. For instance, Thailand has numerous mosquito victims, especially in Buriram, Chaiyaboon, Surin, and Korat. Dengue fever is not usually fatal, but it can make you real sick. In some cases, dengue fever can turn into dengue hemorrhagic fever. This can cause bleeding and even death. Babies and young children are at increased risk of this complication. Because dengue fever is caused by a virus, there is no specific medicine to treat dengue infection. Persons who think they have dengue infection should rest and drink plenty of fluids to prevent dehydration.

How to Avoid Mosquito Bites in the First Place:

Preventing mosquito bites in the first place should be a priority. One of the best natural treatments to avoid mosquito bites is baby oil, methylated spirits, and citronella mixed all together. According to a 2011 French study, consuming alcohol may make your blood tastier for mosquitoes. Men are more likely to be attacked by bugs than women. Another way to be attractive to mosquitos is when you sweating or not taking a shower. When a female mosquito attacks by inserting her proboscis into the flesh, draws blood (food) for the developing eggs. Unfortunately, mosquito bites can also bring diseases or allergic reactions.

Symptoms of Dengue Fever:
High temperature within one week of infection.
Severe headache.
Pain behind the eyes.
Joint and muscle aches.
Metallic taste in the mouth.
Appetite loss.
Abdominal pain.
Nausea and vomiting.
Diarrhea.
Skin rash that appears about four days after the onset of
fever.

Treat Bumps, Blisters, and Warts:

Folliculitis appears when the hair follicle swells up because it's been infected by yeast or bacteria. Blisters are small bubbles filled with fluid and located in the superficial layer of the skin. Warts are raised bumps on your skin (Warts often go away without treatment) caused by the human papillomavirus (HPV). In all these cases the treatment is almost the same. Tea, chamomile bugs, and aloe vera are working very well, but nothing works better than garlic and tomato if you want to treat bumps.

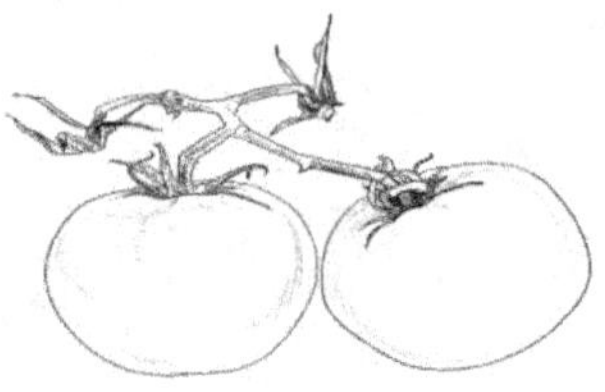

Tomatoes are great for your health as they are a good source of vitamins C, B, E, and potassium. Tomatoes are loaded with a substance called lycopene. Lycopene is an antioxidant that fights free radicals that can damage your immune system. Garlic has a lot of antioxidants and works as an anti-inflammatory with antibacterial properties. Manganese, Phosphorous, Potassium Selenium, vitamins B6, C, and of course the organic sulfur compound allicin that reduces inflammation.

Tomato or Garlic Recipe:

The recipe is the same, in my case I have treated my Blisters with tomato. Both Garlic and Tomato are very effective natural remedies for many health issues, like bacteria, fungi, and infections. Make sure that the Bump, Blister, or Wart is well dried after washing it. Spread fresh melted garlic or a whole tomato directly on the Blister and cover it with a bandage. Do this treatment three times a day for at least 40 minutes. The caustic properties of garlic and tomato will slowly burn the Bump, Blister, or Wart and will be clear after a week. Repeat the process daily.

Peripheral Artery Disease Natural Treatments:

My health journal continues, as I felt some symptoms that need to be checked. Symptoms of poor blood flow like fatigue, numbness, tingling, and a cold feeling in the extremities. So, after a lot of thinking, I end up in a peripheral artery disease doctor. But let's have a look at how we can treat this blood flow disorder with natural remedies.

Stop Smoking:

We all know that smoking restricts blood flow into the extremities. Quitting smoking can return blood flow to normal levels.

Exercise:

Exercise plays a vital role in improving blood circulation.

Ginkgo Biloba:

Ginkgo biloba is well known for its main health benefits associated with improved blood circulation in the body.

Grapeseed Extract:

The grape seed extract is used, as a traditional remedy for conditions related to the heart and blood vessels and poor circulation.

Fish Oil:

Fish oil clean your arteries and helps your blood flow.

Foods Rich in Flavonoids:
Flavonoids which are naturally found in plants and fruits, help as to improving blood circulation.

Massage Therapy:
Improved blood circulation is just one more benefit of massage therapy.

My Ankle-Brachial Index Test Results:

The doctor checked my legs and told me that my blood flow is strong. But he suggests an Ankle-Brachial Index test just to be sure. The nurse took me to a special room and they told me to relax during the test. This test is done by measuring blood pressure at the ankle and in the arm while a person is at rest. My test results were normal. The normal resting ankle-brachial index is 1.0 to 1.4. and means that blood pressure at your ankle is similar to the pressure at your arm. The doctor told me that my symptoms could be caused by a pinched nerve and recommended that I see a chiropractor.

Drug-Induced Psychosis Natural Treatments:

Many people who use drugs have questions like: Can drug-induced psychosis be cured? How long does it last? Can you get Drug-induced psychosis after a single drug experience? Drugs like Marijuana or Methamphetamine can make someone experience temporary symptoms like paranoia. Symptoms are very distressing, but you'll get out of it. Episodes of drug-induced psychosis are common in emergency departments. Many precipitating substances can cause, including Alcohol, Amphetamines, Cannabis, Methamphetamine, Psychedelic drugs, Cocaine, and even Caffeine. After long periods of use, drugs can induce psychotic symptoms that can mimic some serious psychiatric disorders.

A Common Story of Drug-Induced Psychosis:

Some years ago, a friend tried a heavy dose of ice, (methamphetamine or crystal meth). He had a bad trip and start to be paranoid. He was detached and believed that others have hidden motives. He had doubts about the loyalty of his friends and was quickly angry without reason. We were very worried about him. He went to the hospital for two days and the doctors gave him Xanax to calm him down. We all had the same questions:

How Long does Drug-Induced Psychosis Last?

Normally, this kind of psychotic symptom (Transient) can last for a few days until detoxing off the drug and is often characterized by delusions, memory loss, confusion, and sometimes hallucinations. Symptoms of persistent psychosis, on the other hand, can last from three to six months after stopping drug use.

Can you get Drug-Induced Psychosis
After a Single Drug Experience?

It is rare, but yes. You can get transient psychotic symptoms that last for a few days. Persistent psychotic symptoms are often present after substance abuse. People often experience psychotic symptoms with heavy and long-term use or withdrawal.

Can you get Mental Illness After Substance Abuse?

People with a history of psychological disorders, or genetic inheritance together with chronic heavy drug use, can trigger a full-blown psychosis that lasts indefinitely.

Drug-Induced Psychosis Natural Treatments:

Relaxation:

Relax, stop the substance, and find a calm environment.

Natural Herbal Medicines:

Antipsychotic herbs like Brahmi, Panax-ginseng, ginkgo biloba, and anti-anxiety herbs like kava root, gotu kola, saint john plant, and chamomile, can be very helpful.

Nutrition:

Low sugar, low fat, vitamins E and C, melatonin, alpha-lipoic acid, and Omega 3 fatty acids with high EPA.

MEDICAL SURVEYS AND RESEARCH

Medical surveys and health research: Public health research studies for many different diseases. Medical news and health scientific discoveries. You can't treat a disease if you don't know how it behaves. In this chapter, you will find a lot of helpful information about many different diseases.

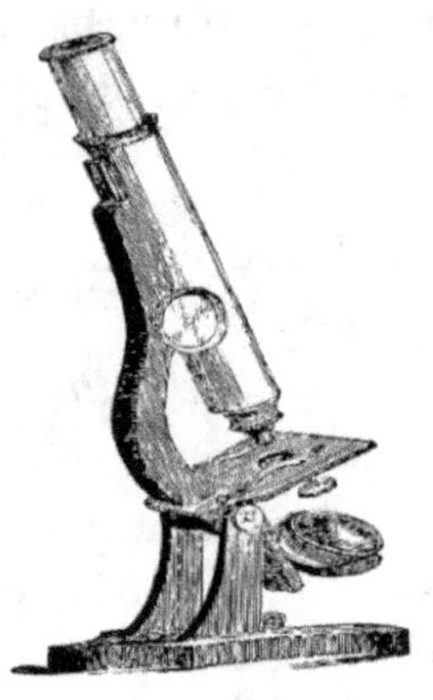

Is Natural Always Good?

Just because something is natural doesn't mean it is always good. Many of the most toxic poisons are plant-based and natural sources. For example, arsenic is poisonous, but this poison grows organically in plants. Another example is Mercury. In my opinion, YES. Nature is always better for health, but only if you know how to use nature. Another example is nicotine (Tobacco) which can be a medicine and a poison at the same time. Finally, to simply prove my point, a natural poison can be harmful in exaggeration, but in small quantities can also be used as a homeopathic remedy!

Are all Chemicals Bad?

Many people think that all chemicals are harmful, but everything in life has two sides. "Chemical" is not a bad word. Chemicals are elements or a combination of elements. Everything in this world is made up of chemical elements. Our human body itself is mixed up with 70% of chemicals which are made up of H_2O molecules! If we analyze a natural product like an apple, we might end up writing a very big list of chemicals. Sometimes synthetic chemicals are good for the environment, as some natural sources are being depleted. Alchemy also uses the knowledge of chemistry, the study of matter by analysis, synthesis, and transmutation. Many of us also know that just because a product is sold at natural foods stores, it doesn't mean that its ingredients are all-natural. So why do they use chemicals? Many times, a synthetic chemical is non-toxic and may be harmless, depending on the usage. A perfect example is a baking soda which is a synthetic chemical (sodium bicarbonate is a natural substance) and harmless. Sodium bicarbonate restores health, cleanses the body, and eradicates toxic substances.

The Dark Side:

It's normal for the public to be suspicious and criticizes any presence of any man-made synthetic chemicals in foods or anywhere else as many of these chemicals often are very toxic or poisonous. Chemicals can be good, bad, and even sometimes evil! Like with any other power on earth, it depends on how you use it. I think that the majority of the things we need may be found in nature, and I hope that people would do more investigation into it and try to uncover its mysteries! Like technology, Man-made chemicals can do more harm than good, especially if we don't know the consequences of chemistry! We must respect and be gentle with chemical elements and not act like we are gods!

Dangers of Mouse Droppings and Urine:

Mouses may carry viruses, bacteria, and other diseases. Diseases are easily spread through mouse droppings and urine. A female house mouse can give birth to more than 50 mice in a single year. One of the most common mouse droppings diseases is a respiratory disease called Hantavirus Pulmonary Syndrome. The majority of cases occur in the spring, when people may breathe in airborne particles. Hantavirus infection in humans may prove fatal. Mouse poop cleaning should be done very carefully, so we can protect ourselves from the transmission of any harmful microorganisms. Cleaning mouse droppings and urine should not be handled without the use of protective gloves and a face mask. A NIEHS study found that the saliva, droppings, or urine of rodents can cause allergies and asthma attacks. Just like being allergic to dogs and cats you can also be allergic to rats and mouses. Mouse droppings, saliva, and urine contain a special type of protein that may cause allergic reactions in sensitive people. People that expose themselves to mice often can develop allergies, even though they have never had them before.

Diseases of Mouse Droppings and Urine:
Hantavirus Pulmonary Syndrome. Rat Bite Fever. Leptospirosis. Encephalomyocarditis. Trichinosis. Bordetellosis. Salmonellosis. Pseudorabies. Swine erysipelas. Toxoplasmosis.

Allergies and Respiratory Diseases:

We separate allergies into food allergies and inhaled allergies. Allergic reactions can cause many strange symptoms. Some Respiratory tract symptoms were observed with food hypersensitivity reactions. In this chapter, you will find a lot of things that you dint know about allergies and asthma.

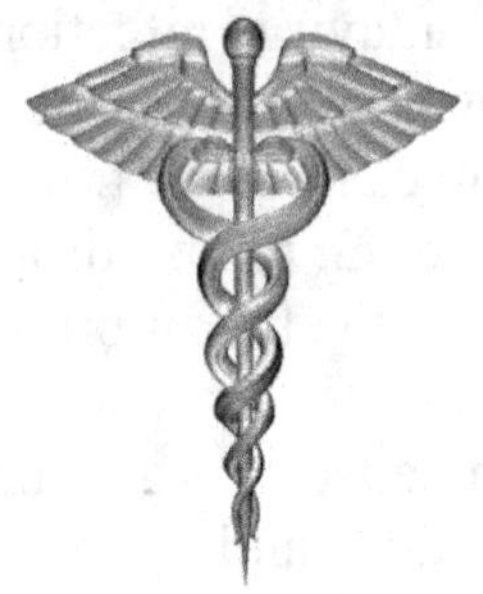

Rhinitis, Acid Reflux, Sinusitis and Asthma:

Long ago, I was in the ENT doctor's office with cold-like symptoms: Runny nose with green thick mucus, difficulty breathing, sneezing, stuffy nose, and mild fever. Were all these symptoms related to my Asthma-GERD disorder? The results were: Allergic rhinitis and sinusitis. I was confused, as I didn't know that there was a connection between rhinitis, acid reflux, sinusitis, and asthma. But first, let's look at all of these diseases and their connections.

Rhinitis and Sinusitis Connection - Rhinosinusitis:

The most common causes of chronic nasal congestion are allergic and nonallergic rhinitis "inflammation of the nose." Non-allergic rhinitis is caused by environmental or occupational irritants. Allergic rhinitis happens when you breathe in something to which you are allergic. Dust, dander, insect venom, and pollen are just a few of the many allergens that can cause allergic rhinitis. Rhinitis and sinusitis can make your life miserable. Recent studies by ENT doctors have better defined the association between rhinitis and sinusitis. Sinusitis is often preceded by rhinitis and rarely occurs without concurrent rhinitis.

Rhinitis-Sinusitis and Asthma Connection:

As we know already, sinusitis is inflammation of the sinuses, which can be acute or chronic and can be caused by infection or by allergies. If you have sinusitis, your symptoms may include pain, sinus discharge, congestion, headache, cough, sore throat, and mild fever. The relationship between sinuses and lower lung airways has been widely noted for decades. People who have asthma are more likely to suffer from chronic sinusitis and patients with sinusitis are much more likely to develop asthma. One of my theories is that post-nasal drainage that commonly caused by rhinitis or sinusitis creates thick mucus that may cause asthma symptoms.

Asthma and Acid Reflux Connection:

Asthma is a disorder that affects the airways. It is caused by inflammation of the airways. It is an incurable disease and symptoms may include coughing, wheezing, chest tightness, and shortness of breath. The severity of the symptoms varies from person to person. Experts say that over half of patients with asthma also have gastroesophageal reflux disease (GERD) and isn't clear why or whether one causes the other.

Acid Reflux and Sinusitis Connection:

Laryngopharyngeal reflux (LPR) and sinusitis, do indeed overlap. Sometimes, the symptoms of GERD can mimic some of the symptoms of sinusitis. The acid reflux causes postnasal drip problems. As a result, sinus infection sticks in the back of the throat. Sinusitis causes all the other symptoms like sinus discharge, headache, congestion, cough, and sore throat!

Rain Allergy: Are you Allergic to Rainwater?

What causes the smell after rain? Do you have a rain allergy? Are your allergies worse in or after a rainstorm? Allergists say that allergies get worse after rain. We already know that rainstorms stir up pollen and that mold and dust mites multiply in humidity. That is a common experience for many people with allergies. Hidden allergens and irritants are a big problem for people with allergies. Thunderstorms and weather changes can trigger asthma attacks. The main asthma triggers are dust mites, mold, pollen, cockroaches, and pets. Because of that, allergy-sufferers must avoid spending time outside on rainy days to minimize exposure to allergens.

Why Does Rain Smell?

The smell after rain can be caused by several things. There is a good rain smell like the one we often notice in the woods, which is caused by bacteria called Actinomycetes, and there is a bad rain smell caused by the acidity of rain, especially in urban environments. Because of pollution, rainwater tends to be more acidic. This kind of rain often causes chemical sensitivities to sensitive people or people with allergies.

Ants Asthma and Respiratory Allergies:
I have had respiratory allergies and sensitivities for many years. Some years ago, I had allergy tests and discovered that I am allergic to dust mites and cockroaches! My allergies are gradually improving following my allergy test, as I am now aware of some of my enemies. I live a healthy lifestyle and I quit smoking. Sometimes, but not often I still get symptoms like stuffy nose, itchy eyes, ear and sinus infections, and even Asthma-like symptoms. Last year I noticed that many of my symptoms happen when Ants were nearby. So, I tried to research but I didn't find so much online! If you search the internet, you will find many studies about the allergic reactions to bites and stings of the Fire Ants, but few have described the direct role of ants in respiratory allergy. I quit the research until I sawed accidentally a new study that suggests that Pharaoh ants can cause allergies and asthma attacks in some sensitive people! Cheol-Woo Kim, MD, Ph.D., and colleagues found that pharaoh ants were responsible for asthma in some patients.

Are Allergies Worse After Trimming Nose Hairs?

When you go to a barbershop in some Asian nations, the barber will start by trimming the hairs on your nose and may even massage your shoulders after cutting your hair. What I noticed was that my allergies worsen after trimming my nose hairs. Nose hair can be very unattractive and annoying, but the purpose of nose hairs is to keep airborne particles from entering the nasal cavity. Nasal hair has a biological purpose. A new study indicated that increased nasal hair density decreases the development of asthma in those suffering from seasonal rhinitis.

Your nose hair contributes to your health in several ways. So before trimming your nose hairs, think twice, because are there for a reason. Nose hairs collect moisture and help to filter the air you breathe so that you are exposed to fewer allergens, such as germs, fungus, and spores.

Blocked Nose After Eating Causes:

Has this ever happened to you? To get a blocked nose after eating food? A blocked nose is very typical for people with allergies. Cold or iced drinks for example slow the cilia in your sinuses. Other foods that you should avoid if you have problems like allergies or sinusitis are alcohol, chocolate, coffee, dairy products, spicy foods, sugar, and yeast. These foods either promote mucus production or promote inflammation. Drinking plenty of water will help to thin the mucus so that it moves more easily. Most of the time the causes of sinusitis are allergic/nonallergic rhinitis or Vasomotor Rhinitis. Vasomotor Rhinitis is chronic rhinitis with the classic symptoms of sneezing and blood vessel congestion of the nasal mucous membranes. For those affected by the condition, the symptoms can be annoying but are not serious. Some examples of common triggers are a dry atmosphere, air pollutants, spicy foods, alcohol, and strong emotions. Any particulate matter in the air, including pollen, dust, mold, or animal dander. Some patients will find that eating (especially, spicy foods) causes more nasal dripping or congestion. Vasomotor rhinitis is not life-threatening.

Hidden Allergy Symptoms:

For sure, allergies can cause sleeping problems, headache, sore throat, increased risk of infections, hives, chronic bronchitis, etc. But what about Vertigo, Nosebleeds, Neck Pain, Mood-Changes, Body Aches, Adrenal Fatigue, and Cold Feet? Can allergies cause all these weird symptoms?

Allergies, Body Aches and Adrenal Fatigue:

Allergies are a major cause of illness all over the world. It is no secret that Sinusitis, Rhinitis, and Asthma go hand to hand. Body aches and pains are common during viral infections, such as colds, but allergies can make you feel miserable too. According to a study, symptoms of allergies often are similar to those of a common cold. Common body symptoms with sinusitis and rhinitis are aches in the neck, back, or legs, together with chronic tiredness, headache, dizziness, and muscle weakness. Fatigue is another common issue with Asthma, rhinosinusitis, and Allergies. The most important reason that asthma, allergies, and chronic rhinosinusitis can trigger fatigue, is your body's oxygen levels. Breathlessness is the sensation of not getting enough air, as a result, you get low oxygen levels in your body. When oxygen levels are too low, your body doesn't have the power to operate correctly. Normal activities like exercise with lower oxygen levels can cause a lack of sleep and chronic fatigue syndrome in people with breathing issues.

Allergies, Histamines and Adrenal Fatigue:

Adrenal glands sit in pairs at the top of each kidney. Adrenal fatigue is any decrease in the ability of the adrenal glands to carry out their normal functions. Histamines are important parts of the human body, but they can easily become a source of chronic inflammation. When we are under stress or having an allergy attack, our body stimulates the release of antibodies, which attach themselves to mast cells as a result, histamine is released from the mast cells. The more histamine released, the more cortisol it takes to control the inflammatory response. That, unfortunately, can lead to adrenal fatigue and larger allergic reactions. Histamine tends to react to practically anything from taste, feelings, touch, and smell.

Can Allergies Cause Vertigo?

Vertigo is a sense of rotation like the world is spinning. It is caused by balance disorders and many health conditions like medications, a dysfunction in the inner ear, or (less common) from the brain. There are many different causes of vertigo, but the most common is benign paroxysmal positional vertigo (BPPV). In this article, we will research two less common causes and the links and connections between Allergies, and vertigo.

The Link Between Allergies and Vertigo:

For sure, there is a link between Allergies and Dizziness, but what about vertigo? Several conditions can cause you to feel dizzy or nauseous. For sure, GERD and allergies are some of them. The strong connection between LPR, Allergies, and postnasal drip is real. All those symptoms often affect your middle ear and the back of your throat. Ear pain is often a symptom of an ear infection or sinus infection.

Middle ear pressure changes, such as allergies can cause swelling of the Eustachian tube or the presence of fluid in the middle ear. So YES, Allergies can cause vertigo!

Allergies and Nosebleeds Connection:

Rhinitis is a condition where the inside of the nose becomes inflamed. Allergic and nonallergic rhinitis or mixed rhinitis is inflammation of our nostrils caused by viruses, bacteria, irritants, or allergens.

Can Rhinitis or Allergies Cause Bloody Nose?

Usually, symptoms come and go and can be annoying. Bloody noses are common with Rhinitis because the lining of the nose, which has many blood vessels, is constantly irritated. For me, it happens most of the time in the morning, when my nose gets dry. Another reason is that the lining of the nose is itchy and is often rubbed or scratched. Nosebleeds are a common problem for people who have allergies but, most of the time these nosebleeds don't cause any serious health problems.

Allergies Cold Feet and Hands:

Allergens are what trigger a series of reactions by the immune system during an allergic reaction. Chronic allergies can cause cold hands and feet. An allergy can lower your blood pressure, which will finally cause cold hands and feet. One of the bigger problems of asthma is that it can trigger blood pressure. Low blood pressure is one of the main signs that an asthma attack is occurring. During an asthma attack, bronchioles constrict and air cannot pass through them as freely.

Can Allergies Cause Neck Pain?

Neck pain is discomfort in any of the structures in the neck. Many conditions can cause chronic neck pain. Allergies, acid reflux and headaches are all related. The link between migraines and allergies is caused by sinusitis or by a chemical reaction to an allergen, which annoys the blood vessels. Tension and stress may lead to neck pain. Other factors that may play an important role together with allergies are •Continuous working for a long time. •Certain foods can cause sensitivity. •Position of working (While in the office or when working on your computer). •Changes in sleep or lack of sleep. •Stress. •Poor posture.

Can Allergies Affect your Mood?

How can allergies affect your mood or energy level? Most of us when thinking about allergies, we think of some typical symptoms such as sneezing, itchy eyes, shortness of breath and nausea. But did you know that food, seasonal and chemical allergies (which are the reaction of the immune system) can create emotional symptoms like anxiety, irritability, compulsions, confusion, palpitations, sweating, trembling, inability to concentrate, or mental fog? In the middle of the twentieth century, asthma and allergy were often seen as psychosomatic illnesses.

Conclusion: Food chemicals and seasonal allergies can cause mental symptoms in some sensitive persons. Stress can also affect allergic reactions. Allergies attack your immune system and this happens without you even noticing it. A weakened immune system will increase your anxiety.

Dust Mites and Sinusitis Connection:

We spoke before about the connection between Rhinitis and Sinusitis. Dust mites and sinusitis are like bread and butter. House dust mites are tiny (up to 0.3 mm) animals related to spiders and live on mattresses, bedding, carpets, and curtains. The number of mites can be reduced, but cannot be eliminated. Mites' feces contain particular proteins that can trigger an allergy in sensitive people. Sinusitis is an infection or inflammation of the sinuses. Conditions that can cause sinus blockage include the common cold, rhinitis, and allergic rhinitis. Our mucous membranes form a physical barrier against bacteria and viruses. Dust mites can cause a lot of problems to the mucous membranes. Mucous membranes make the immune system overreact and cause rhinitis and Sinusitis.

How to Stop Dust Mites:

Microfibers: This is one of the few times that synthetic materials have proven useful. Microfiber bedding can be used to completely stop dust mites. Good quality Microfibers can be used as an external barrier to allergens and therefore cannot be colonized by mites. Studies showed that people can now remove mite allergens from their home environment! Unfortunately, microfibers are made from polyester and nylon (polyamide), which are made from petroleum. Polyester is a synthetic fiber derived from carbon, air, water, and oil.

Organic cotton and latex: Many other natural fabrics can stop dust mites and are ideal for blocking other allergens. For example, all-Cotton with tightly woven 100% mattresses and bedsheets can eliminate exposure to dust mites. Organic cotton is natural, and no pesticides or other harmful chemicals are used. Latex is also naturally resistant to dust mites.

Latex naturally repels dust mites. I use a cervical pillow with 100% organic latex for my neck problems and cotton satin sheets.

Lip - Eyes Twitching and Sinusitis Connection:

We all know that Sinusitis and headaches are connected. If you have sinusitis and migraine, it's probably because of your Sinus. But what about lip-twitching and eyes-twitching? We all know that these kinds of symptoms are alarming.

Eyes Twitching and Sinusitis Connection:

Blepharospasm is an involuntary spasm of the muscles in the eyelid. The eyes are very near to sinuses and can get affected when sinuses have inflammation. Some nerves of your eyes are passing through your sinuses and ending up in your brain. When your sinuses are inflamed, some nerves can get irritated and cause muscle spasms.

Lip Twitching and Sinusitis Connection:

It's something that can happen to anyone and can affect your top, bottom, or both lips and is very common. It can happen by many things including stress or fatigue, deficiency of potassium, lack of electrolytes, withdrawal, or excess intake of alcohol, drugs, or cigarettes. Sometimes lip twitching can also be caused by neck pain. Lip twitching, in most cases, is self-limiting. Another common cause is sinusitis. Irritated sinuses around your eyes and nose can put pressure on the facial nerve.

Multiple Chemical Sensitivities Syndrome:
Both chemical sensitivities and allergies can invoke an immune system response. Irritants such as pollution and cigarette smoke worsen conditions such as asthma. I had a lot of food and chemical sensitivities in the past. One example was my sensitivity to mosquito coil. Many people that are sensitive to mosquito coil get shortness of breath every time they are nearby. According to studies, using a coil is equivalent to smoking 130 cigarettes. Mosquito coils can cause liver and cornea damage, asthma symptoms, headaches, and lightheadedness. Some sensitivities are not true allergies, but the terms allergy and sensitivity are often used interchangeably. Multiple chemical sensitivities syndrome is when an individual has symptoms in response to certain man-made chemicals. This chemical sensitivity is also called "environmental illness". One thing is for sure high doses of chemicals make people sick.

Multiple Chemical Sensitivities Syndrome Treatment:
There are no effective or proven treatments. Eliminate chemicals that cause chemical sensitivities and find replacements with natural alternatives. Chemical avoidance is the secret to a better life. Another way to fight your chemical sensitivities is by getting stronger. A strong immune system can fight back any disease. I recommend exercise, good organic food, vitamins and fasting detoxification.

Multiple Chemical Sensitivities Triggers and Causes:
It is not clear what causes the symptoms of chemical sensitivity in some individuals. Researchers believe that caused by systemic damage from toxins. Here are some triggers: Petroleum-based products. Agricultural chemicals. Industrial cleaning chemicals. Formaldehyde and aldehyde.

Glues. Varnishes. Polishes. Paints. Mosquito coil. Insect repellents. Laundry detergents. Perfumes, (lotion, after-shave lotion, nail polish). Air-fresheners. Shampoos. Gasoline (petrol) or diesel fuel.

Asthma Symptoms Hours After Exercise:

Do you have asthma symptoms hours after exercise? Exercise-induced asthma is very common. EIA may begin during exercise (typically within 10/15 minutes) or after the exercise. Some individuals may experience delayed bronchoconstriction (late phase response) four to twelve hours after completing an exercise. This late-phase response is related more to inflammatory changes. Inflammation is a term used in medicine to describe how the body reacts to various types of injury or irritation or infection. It's important to say that in some people, asthma is not causing any symptoms, such as cough or wheezing.

Asthma or GERD? Some people with exercise-induced asthma feel tired, or dizzy after exercising and some may even experience a stomach ache. That's one of the reasons that 70 percent of all people with asthma also have GERD. About 70% of asthmatics also have allergies. As a result, the late phase response of Asthma symptoms may be due to acid reflux. Sometimes when we workout, we press our abdomen muscles without we noticed and after a heavy or late at night meal, the symptoms start to occur. LPR or airway reflux (silent reflux) can also be the problem.

Dehydration and Asthma:

The link between dehydration and asthma remains a medical mystery. Asthma is a chronic and serious condition. Symptoms include a cough, wheezing, chest tightness, and breathlessness, and can vary in severity from person to person. Research today seeks to uncover some of the mysteries around the illness. 75 percent of the population has some degree of dehydration, significant enough to affect their health. Asthma attacks are often linked to airborne allergens, respiratory infections, exercise, cold air that enters the lungs, stress, and gastroesophageal reflux disease.

Is Dehydration Bad for Asthmatics?

One new theory suggests that asthma is caused mostly by dehydration in the body. Dr. F. Batmanghelidj, the author of ABC of Asthma, Allergies, and Lupus, says that asthma, allergies, and other health problems are directly related to chronic dehydration. Mostly all of the asthma triggers cause dehydration which leads to shortness of breath. Stress and strong emotions, exercise, hot or cold air blowing air, and so on. Because of allergies, many people breathe through the mouth. If you breathe through your mouth for a long time your mouth will get dry. Drinking two to three cups of water and putting a pinch of sea salt on the tongue are the best treatments for bronchospasm, which can be brought on by dehydration.

Dehydration Symptoms: Dark yellow or orange urine. Infrequent urination. Reduced sweat. Thirst. Dry mouth/nose. Dizziness. Weakness. Overheating.

Dehydration Treatment: Prevent dehydration by drinking fluids frequently. Eat hydrating foods, such as fresh fruits and vegetables. Avoid Alcohol and caffeine. Avoid Exercise when is hot. Drink Chamomile tea and consume coconut water, which is high in electrolytes.

Asthma and Poor Circulation:

Asthma gets worse when temperature and weather changes occur. Cold is one of the biggest triggers. Rapid weather changes can cause an asthma attack to occur.

Feeling Cold with Asthma:

One of the main reasons that you may feel cold or that you have cold hands or feet in chronic asthma is that your body is just exhausted. Another part of the reason is that during an attack, many asthmatics will hyperventilate and raise their oxygen levels because their lungs are working so hard. Cold hands or feet in asthma, can be a symptom that blood isn't going to your peripheral body areas. Health research suggests that cold hands and feet are a classical symptom of chronic hyperventilation.

Asthma and Poor Circulation:

Poor circulation is a common symptom that occurs in people with chronic diseases and the most common cause of poor circulation is low CO_2 in the arterial blood. Poor circulation is another classic symptom of over-breathing.

Asthma and Hypoxia:

Several causes can lead to hyperventilation and one of them is Hypoxia. Hyperventilation and mountain sickness are connected.

Shortness of Breath After Quit Smoking:

Do you experience shortness of breath after quitting smoking? You are not alone. The health benefits start 20 minutes after your last cigarette, but kicking a long-term habit does not happen overnight. Your body is addicted to nicotine and it takes 72 hours after you quit smoking for the nicotine to be out of your body. You may face several nicotine withdrawal symptoms. Withdrawal symptoms begin shortly after quitting and then rapidly increase in intensity until they peak. Many people with asthma will get asthma symptoms after quitting smoking. That is because the lungs are repairing themselves, and the cilia (little hairs inside your lungs) are growing back. This makes your chest feel itchy and a feeling like you are not breathing properly. Another theory says that stress is also a trigger for shortness of breath. Quitting smoking can cause anxiety and your chest muscles can get tense which makes you feel like you can't breathe. Another thing is that at least one of the chemicals in cigarettes acts as a bronchodilator that actually relieves asthma symptoms, but in the long term, it damages your lungs.

Withdrawal Symptoms List:

Irritability and Aggression. Mild Depression. Restlessness. Poor concentration. Increased appetite. Light-headedness. Insomnia. Shortness of breath. Constipation. Coughing with mucous. Sore throat. Gaseous Stomach. Fatigue. Heartburn. Smoking tobacco is both a physical addiction and a psychological habit. The lungs come equipped with a self-cleaning cycle. The day you quit, your body starts to recover. Cleaning your lungs after quitting smoking is one of the smartest things you should do. After quitting smoking, it is important to help the lungs rebuild. Many people who smoked heavily for years assume that they are no longer at risk after quitting, but unfortunately, that's not the truth. Whether you're a teen smoker or a lifetime 2 pack–a–day smoker, after quitting smoking efforts must be made to repair the lungs from the damage and scarring of smoking.

Clean your Lungs Faster After Quitting Smoking:

Try to avoid second-hand smoke and carbon monoxide to prevent further damage. Pineapple (Bromelain), ginger, horseradish, avocado, and rosemary have healing effects on the lungs. Start to exercise with small steps and gradually increase what you do over time. Drink about eight glasses of water daily and try to eat plenty of fiber and veggies. Breathing and relaxation exercises are also very good for repairing the lungs.

GERD - LPR - Gastritis - H Pylori:

In this chapter, We will solve the puzzle between shortness of breath, GERD – Acid Reflux, and LPR, as I found out that all these diseases coexist. Asthma is most often caused by an allergy or by irritants that get into breathing passages. It is estimated that over half of patients with asthma also have gastroesophageal reflux disease (GERD). Asthma and acid reflux often occur together. It isn't clear why or whether one causes the other, but acid reflux can worsen asthma and asthma can worsen acid reflux. In my case, I think asthma came first. When I was a kid, I was diagnosed with Asthmatic-bronchitis.

Breathing Problems, Acid Reflux and LPR:

Unfortunately, some asthma drugs can worsen acid reflux. Asthma doctors will drive some tests to measure your lung function, like Spirometry, but most of them will never ask you if you have GERD or any other abdomen issues. Gastroesophageal reflux disease is when stomach acids, food, and fluids flow back into the esophagus. Acid reflux can irritate the food pipe. Untreated chronic GERD can cause inflammation of the esophagus. As I mentioned before, GERD causes shortness of breath and happens mostly every time we are bloated. Some of the reasons are poor digestion and gas together with esophagitis. Bloating can lead to shortness of breath and restrict the movement of the diaphragm. When you can't take, a deep breath can lead to swallowing air (aerophagia). Just be aware that according to some studies, Gastroesophageal reflux disease may cause pulmonary diseases. Another possible reason is that during a reflux attack, stomach acid that creeps into the esophagus can enter the lungs. Finally, another reason for the shortness of breath can be excess mucus or gastric fluids in the back of the throat. Glands in the lining of the esophagus produce mucus and if you have a problem with the muscles of the lower esophageal sphincter can cause symptoms like excess phlegm/gastric fluids, cough, and pain with swallowing.

Laryngeal-Pharyngeal Reflux:

Symptoms of LPR are often not typical gastroesophageal reflux disease (GERD) symptoms. Laryngopharyngeal reflux and GERD are two related, yet different, disease states. Laryngeal-pharyngeal reflux is common in asthmatics. In my case, I had asthma symptoms together with sinus infections, laryngitis, and other upper respiratory issues. For many patients, if they get their reflux under control the asthma symptoms also disappear. Laryngopharyngeal reflux is sometimes called "silent reflux." Many patients fail to recognize this association because the classic symptoms of acid reflux, heartburn, and regurgitation, may be absent. ***Conclusion***: Asthma, GERD and allergies, acid reflux, and LPR often occur together. Try to treat your asthma, and if you have your acid reflux under control then your asthma symptoms will also disappear. Find natural ways to cure both. Keep your diet healthy.

Hidden LPR - Airway Reflux,
the Unknown Enemy:

As I mentioned earlier, LPR is a condition that occurs in a person who has gastroesophageal reflux disease (GERD). In the case of silent reflux, the stomach acid not only rises the esophagus but makes it all the way up into the larynx or the pharynx. Hidden airway reflux is difficult to diagnose. Researchers believe that up to 40% of the population has LPR, but it goes undiagnosed for decades. Many Doctors misdiagnose LPR disease and confuse LPR with allergies, sinusitis, and asthma. Did you know that asthma is one of the most common misdiagnoses because silent reflux mimics asthma? Many young adults have Airway Reflux but go undiagnosed for their whole lives.

(Undiagnosed LPR) My Personal Experience:

I had asthma when I was a kid. Doctors don't know which comes first GERD or asthma. I had stomach issues as a teenager, but they were mostly caused by dairy consumption. One day after a strong coffee, I had my first gastritis attack. I had dizziness, an upset stomach, and shortness of breath, but without abdominal pain, so I didn't know what it was, and because of the shortness of breath I thought that was an asthma attack. Long story short, I had these attacks once or two times a year. The first thing I did was to visit a Pulmonologist. After some tests and spirometry, he told me that I have mild allergic asthma. But I was still concerned because something seemed off about this doctor's diagnosis. Finally, one day after a severe gastritis attack, I went immediately for an endoscopy, and the doctor diagnosed me with gastritis, GERD-LPR, and esophagitis. All these years, my LPR and gastritis worsen my asthma. Normally, when acid reflux occurs, Acid and Pepsin are released from the stomach and travel as fluid, but often in the case of LPR, aspirated into the throat, nose, mouth, ears, and lungs. Pepsin is a very useful enzyme that helps the stomach break down proteins. Outside the stomach, it causes damage to cells and inflammation.

Symptoms of Hidden Airway Reflux:
•Mild hoarseness. •Sensation of a lump in the throat. •Chronic cough. •Asthma and apnea. •Sensation of mucous sticking in the throat and a need to clear the throat. •Post-nasal drip. •Difficulty swallowing. •Sore throat. *Other symptoms are:*

Cold Sensation in the Throat when Inhaling:
Gastric acid travels into the esophagus and exceeds the usual limit. If you have LPR, you can suddenly get a cold feeling in your throat without any apparent reason and you will wonder why. With acid reflux, acids travel from the stomach and rise into the esophagus to irritate the vocal cord. As a result, you get a symptom of vocal cord dysfunction. You may feel like you have inhaled toothpaste after brushing your teeth. Many people that suffer from silent reflux have this symptom and don't know the reason.

Breathing Spasms (Hiccups):
Most of the time kids with GERD have this symptom, but also some adults. Unfortunately, there is not so much info out there about this symptom.

LPR Reflux and Teeth Problems:

Can Gerd and LPR cause teeth problems? The short answer is YES. Patients with acid reflux are at greater risk of periodontal problems. Gerd and especially LPR Reflux can cause teeth problems. If you have chronic acid reflux, it's not only your esophagus that you should be worried about. The stomach acid goes up into the esophagus and can ultimately get to the mouth. Because of acid, most LPR patients have symptoms like a metallic taste and dry mouth, which intensify plaque and dental bacteria and that can cause teeth problems like gum disease. *Symptoms Of Tooth Decay Due To Acid Reflux:* Pain or irritation in your mouth. Sensitivity to certain foods and drinks, especially hot and cold. Sharp tooth edges. Thinning or shortened teeth. Darkening teeth.

LPR and Vocal Cord Dysfunction Connection:

Vocal cord dysfunction or paradoxical vocal fold motion is abnormal adduction of the vocal cords. The vocal cords normally open up when you breathe in and out, but with VCD, vocal cords are closing. Vocal cord dysfunction can be very hard to detect. The discovery of VCD disease is quite new (1951). Vocal Cord Dysfunction is sometimes confused with asthma because has similar triggers and symptoms and in some cases, it is wrong-treated with inhaled or systemic corticosteroids. On the other hand, many people with asthma also have VCD.

What can Cause Vocal Cord Dysfunction?

Many patients diagnosed with VCD have also acid reflux which irritates the throat. So, the prime cause of VCD is gastroesophageal reflux disease (GERD) and LPR-airway reflux. Studies found that vocal cord dysfunction and GERD connection are strong. Other causes are exposure to inhaled allergens, emotional stress, postnasal drip, exercise, and neurological conditions. Doctors in the 19th century were so convinced that asthma was a psychological disorder, today some blinded studies try to emphasize anxiety as a primary cause while more recent research indicates a likely physical etiology. As a result, or as planned, some people with VCD use anti-anxiety drugs and have harmful side effects without reason. The best treatments for VCD are natural. First, you must treat any underlying conditions such as gastroesophageal reflux disease (GERD) and LPR airway reflux, allergies, or sinusitis, and then you must learn some breathing and Speech techniques. Symptoms can include shortness of breath, a feeling of tightness in the throat or chest, frequent clearing your throat or cough, hoarse voice, wheezing, voice changes, a feeling of choking.

Helicobacter Pylori:

Has this ever happened to you? Feeling that something is wrong with your body, even if most doctors say you're fine? Have you ever had symptoms like Acid reflux, diarrhea, gas, heartburn, mild fever, anxiety, fatigue, and nausea? If the answer to all these questions is yes, then welcome to H. pylori infection. H. pylori and its effects on the human body are still very poorly understood. Helicobacter pylori can disrupt the mucous lining of the stomach allowing a stomach ulcer to form. Lifestyle factors, such as alcohol abuse, physical and emotional stress, unhealthy eating habits, and smoking, cause peptic ulcers and gastritis. More than 60% of the world's population is known to be infected with Helicobacter pylori, usually acquired in childhood. Is passed from person to person in a variety of ways. Kissing is one of those ways (passed through saliva) as well as unsanitary conditions in food or water. Helicobacter pylori can cause many different symptoms, but most people infected with the bacteria never have symptoms or problems at all. If H. pylori start to make symptoms, visit a doctor for diagnosis and tests. The bacteria can also attach to cells of the stomach, causing stomach inflammation (Gastritis) or peptic ulcer and can stimulate the production of excess stomach acid (G.E.R.D).

Symptoms of Helicobacter Pylori:

Heartburn/Acid Reflux. Diarrhea/Constipation/Gas/Bloating. Fatigue and Low Energy. Nausea & Vomiting. Unexplained Weight Loss. Mood-changes/Anxiety. Bad Breath. Sinus Problems. Chills/joint pain. Frequent urination. Mild-Fever.

Helicobacter Pylori Treatment:

The H. pylori treatment is triple-drug therapy, a mix of two antibiotics and one antacid for two weeks. Doctors will recommend also a diet or stop smoking if you do and stop drinking alcohol. Remember that taking a high dose of antibiotics can also destroy your good bacteria, so it's always a good idea to take probiotic supplements.

How Long does it Take to Cure H Pylori with Antibiotics?

Symptoms should begin to subside within a few days. The antibiotics can irritate your stomach, so it may take a week or two before the GERD subsides. Normally you must go back to the hospital after a month for breath or stool tests to see if you are still infected. Once the H. pylori bacteria are gone from your body, the chance of being infected again is very low.

H pylori and Neurological Symptoms:

Arthritis, and fibromyalgia. Helicobacter Pylori can cause Neurological symptoms by preventing stomach acid production, which leads to vitamin B12 and mineral deficiency. Individuals with H pylori and gastritis may develop pernicious Anemia. H. Pylori infection can lead to some forms of arthritis, fibromyalgia syndrome symptoms, and neurological symptoms like numbness and paresthesias. Any problem that you might have could be due to H pylori infection.

Helicobacter Pylori Best Test:

My Personal Experience with the Test:
So, I went back to the hospital today to find out if I have helicobacter pylori. I did some research before going to the hospital to determine the most accurate test for H pylori. Believe it or not, most doctors out there are not aware of which test is the most accurate. Let's determine now which Helicobacter pylori test is the most effective.

Helicobacter Pylori Best Test:
There are four different types of H. pylori tests…
•Blood Antibody Test. •Stool Antigen Test. •Urea Breath Test. •Stomach Biopsy Test.

Blood Antibody Test:
Unfortunately, the blood antibody test will show positive traces of H. pylori, even long after the bacterium has been treated successfully. So is not a good idea to use an H. pylori blood test after you have been treated!

Stomach Biopsy Test:
The stomach biopsy test is not only costly, but also frightening for the majority of us. During an endoscopy, you lie on your side and a thin tube with a camera is passed down to your esophagus and into your stomach. Endoscopy is fantastic if you want to identify stomach and duodenal ulcers or gastritis, but if you just want to see if the bacterium is there, is not the best test.

Urea Breath Test:

The urea breath test is a very expensive test and is not always available, but the most important is that the results are often inconsistent.

Stool Antigen Test:

This is the most accurate test for H Pylori. A stool culture is used to detect the presence of pathogenic bacteria and help to diagnose an infection. A stool test is the best test for H pylori, as it is inexpensive, it's easy, and you just need to provide a stool sample.

Can Gas Cause Chest Pain?

People that suffer from IBS (irritable bowel syndrome), ulcerative colitis, GERD, gallbladder disease, and Gastritis are suffering also from trapped stomach gases. High fiber foods, artificial sweeteners, carbonated drinks, like soda, and certain sugary or dairy foods can cause a lot of gas. Sometimes gas accumulated in the abdomen and stretches the muscles of the food pipe and the nerve endings. As a result, gas makes you feel breathless as it requires more effort for your lungs to expand. It isn't uncommon for chest gas pains to be severe enough to make people think they're experiencing a heart attack. Many people with gas symptoms end up in hospitals to see if they had a heart attack. This extreme discomfort causes anxiety and anxiety just make the symptoms worse.

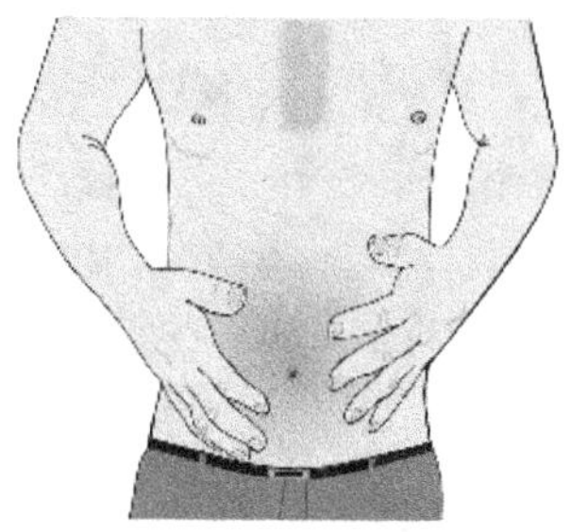

How you Know it is Gas and not a Heart Attack?
Here are some Symptoms of Trapped Gas:
Heaviness and high pressure in the chest area.
Belching and bloating of the abdomen.
Sweating and panic.
Sharp pains in the abdominal area.
Shortness of breath.
Absence of appetite.
Feeling better while walking.

Symptoms of a Heart Attack:
Chest pain - A sensation of pressure, tightness in the center of your chest. Pain that spreads to the arms, neck, jaw, or back.
Feeling dizzy or having nausea. Shortness of breath. A feeling of anxiety. Weakness and tiredness. Back pain or pressure.

Do not Fight your Symptoms:

There are so many scary symptoms like Chills, fever, paresthesia, dizziness, dry mouth, sleepiness, shortness of breath, weakness, ear ringing, anorexia, weight loss, fatigue, swelling, arrhythmia, chest pain, hearing loss, sore throat, abdominal pain, bloating, constipation or diarrhea, heartburn, nausea and so on…

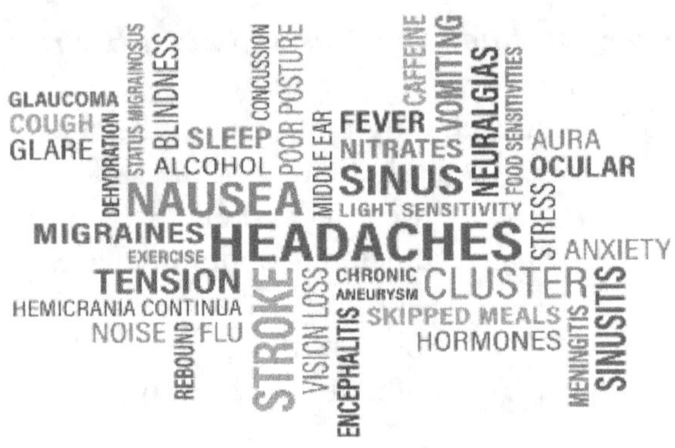

In reality, nobody likes symptoms, as in most cases are annoying and a result of a disease, but believe it or not, symptoms are not the enemy. Symptoms are a signal that our body sends that something is wrong. Also, what is more important is that our body heals and repairs itself. Today, unfortunately, doctors do not fight the cause but the symptom. Do a favor to yourself, research and treat the cause, not the symptom. Doctors give medicines such as antibiotics and steroids that in reality make you sicker, only to calm down the symptoms. For example, in ancient times, people knew the benefit of sneezing and used to sneeze on purpose. We sneeze because our lymphatic system tries to clean out toxins, bacteria, and viruses. Also, a sneeze is so powerful that suppressing it can cause nose-bleeds and damage blood vessels. Another symptom is fever. Fever's purpose is to raise the body's temperature to eliminate viruses and bacteria that are sensitive to temperature changes. Coughing is also another way in which our body gets rid of foreign particles like bacteria, microbes, irritants, and mucus. Hiccups most of the time, come after eating or drinking too much or too quickly. High blood pressure as another example, is a sign of stress in the body and can increase the risk of stroke and heart disease. We feel pain because our nerves send messages to our brains about what's going on. Arrhythmias may be a sign of electrolyte imbalances, changes in your heart muscle, or even a sign of coronary artery disease. The list can go on and on, but the answer is simple, just listen to your body and treat yourself the right way, fight the cause, not the symptom.

Physical Diseases and Panic Attacks:

What they don't want you to Know: Physical diseases can cause panic attacks: Diabetes, Overactive thyroid, Gerd, Rhinitis, Asthma, and Irritable bowel syndrome (IBS). Yes, if that is the case, you may have more than one or two panic attacks a year and not have a panic disorder. Media and some websites spread fear, and as a result, people visit psychiatrists and become victims of the pharmaceutical industry. For example, the thyroid gland is one of the largest endocrine glands and it is found in the neck right below Adam's apple. Hypothyroidism more commonly causes depression and fatigue. Now, on the other hand, Hyperthyroidism, which is when too much of the thyroid hormone is produced can cause panic attacks.

The Link Between GERD and Panic Attacks:

Studies found that GERD increases anxiety and depression and creates a vicious cycle. Anxiety increase symptoms of GERD and GERD can increase anxiety. The acid irritates your airways, especially if you have LPR (silent reflux). When bile refluxes into the stomach, the stomach secretes acid in an attempt to neutralize the bile and can cause bloating, heartburn, chest tightness, difficulty swallowing, sinusitis, laryngitis, or even an asthma attack. Acid touches the nerves in your esophagus. Esophagus reflux can also cause symptoms that one does during an allergic reaction. Are that enough symptoms to get panic? The solution is simple. If you eliminate your symptoms of GERD with natural ways like nutrition and exercise you will break this vicious cycle. Unfortunately, Psychiatrists do not tend to link gastroesophageal reflux (GERD) and irritable bowel syndrome (IBS) with anxiety and panic and usually misdiagnose patients. Keep in mind that an Acid reflux attack can be triggered by many things including exercise, stress, cold weather, bad food habits, lying in the bed with a full stomach, caffeine, and so on. Yes, even exercise can make acid reflux temporarily worse, but in the long term, it helps a lot with GERD. ***Conclusion***: Physical diseases can cause panic attacks. Diseases like diabetes, GERD, overactive thyroid, rhinitis, asthma, and irritable bowel syndrome (IBS) can be your hidden cause. So please run some tests to find out if any of these diseases is the cause before visiting a psychiatrist.

Gum Disease and Tooth Infections:

Without a doubt, oral diseases can affect the overall health status of a patient. Periodontitis has been associated with several systemic conditions. Many other conditions can be affected such as cardiovascular disease, diabetes, and respiratory infections. This time, we will focus only on the most common interactions and adverse effects:

Can Gum Disease Cause Mouth Ulcers?

A week ago, I went on a business trip and forgot to brush my sensitive teeth and gums. As a result, I had some gum pain. Two days later, after I ate a sweet dessert, I felt ulcers and canker sores on my mouth and lips. A question came to my mind straight away, can gum disease and periodontitis cause mouth ulcers and canker sores? Canker sores are usually small ulcers with a white or gray center and begin as a red spot or bump. Mouth ulcers, in general, occur inside the mouth and are bacterial. Periodontitis, or gum disease, is a condition in which the gums and periodontal structures become inflamed. Both gum diseases, gingivitis, and periodontitis can cause inflammation and gum bleeding with other symptoms like difficulty chewing, dry mouth, bad breath, swollen, tender gums, and a sour taste in the mouth. If you ever notice any of these symptoms, find soon as possible your dentist for an appointment. Swollen gums and canker sores can be treated with proper oral hygiene and the right diet.

Can a Tooth Infection Cause Sinus Problems?

Many times, people with sinus problems have also hidden gum disease. How can you tell if it's a dental abscess or a sinus problem? Bacteria in your mouth can build up and eventually cause tooth infections. If an upper infected tooth has roots that have extended into the sinus can lead to sinusitis. According to Dr. Peterson, tooth infections cause 10 percent of all sinusitis. Many conditions such as nasal polyps, allergies, or tooth infections can lead to sinus infections. A bad tooth can cause many health problems like sinus infections, chest infections, colds, and so on. Bad teeth can cause these problems because they can send infected bacteria to your body. Tooth infections don't always announce themselves with a toothache. Just remember the longer you leave it untreated, the more difficult it will be.

Dizziness After Dental Work, is it Normal?

Do you feel dizzy after dental work? Can dental work cause dizziness or even vertigo? Recently I went to the dentist to clean my teeth. The dentist tried to remove the plaque and tartar from above and below the gum line. After a half-hour of a hard job, the doctor told me to stand up. But when I stand up, I felt dizziness and lightheadedness. That was a new experience for me. So, I decided to research and I found that this dizziness was a common thing. The short answer is yes, it's normal. Especially if you have had a lot of work done at this appointment. Some people even experience vertigo. Vertigo is a type of dizziness often described as a Spinning sensation in the head. Vertigo is a sense of extreme dizziness and loss of balance.

So, What Cause the Dizziness?

1) Getting up after a long lying position in the dental chair can lead to dizziness for some people. You may experience low blood pressure when you suddenly move from a lying position to an upright position. 2) Dental experience causes excessive stress. 3) Tooth anesthetic can also cause dizziness. Conclusion: Dizziness after dental work is considered normal most of the time. If you feel dizzy, eat well and rest.

Can Sciatica Cause Neck Pain?

Can back pain like sciatica cause neck or arms problems? Sciatica is just a symptom, not a disease. The most common reason for sciatica is Lumbar Spinal Stenosis, but eventually, many other diseases can cause sciatica, like Piriformis syndrome and Osteophytes. For many years after my motorcycle accident, I wondered what the connection might be between lower back pain (sciatica) and neck problems with numbness in the hands or tingling. For many years, I looked for an answer, but I couldn't find anything. As most of the time, cervical and lumbar radiculopathy are not connected. On my Facebook feed one day, I came upon a Dr. Axe article about Piriformis disease. Then I started to research and I found out that Piriformis syndrome and Osteophytes can cause arm and neck problems.

Piriformis Syndrome:

Piriformis is located in the buttock region and is a condition in which piriformis muscle irritates the sciatic nerve and causes pain, numbness, and tingling in the leg and foot. My Piriformis syndrome started after my motorbike accident, My surgical plate has a screw that pressing this muscle, as you can see in the picture. I didn't know until now that this syndrome was responsible for my weird symptoms.

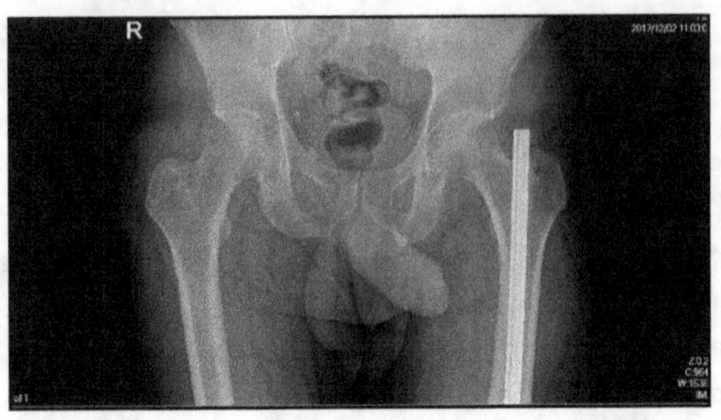

Piriformis syndrome Symptoms:

•A dull ache in the buttock. •Reduced range of motion of the hip joint. •Pain and irritation of the sciatic nerve (sciatica). •Tingling or numbness in the lower body. •Increased pain after too much sitting. •Sometimes neck pains and headaches. •Stomach Pain and Constipation.

Osteophytes:

This disease can be asymptomatic for several years. Osteophytes are bony projections that form along joint margins. Bone spurs develop in areas of injury or inflammation.

Symptoms of Osteophytes:

•Compression of the sciatic nerve •Unexpected muscle weakness •Chronic lower back pain. •Burning or tingling in the hands or feet. •Muscle spasms or cramps. •Radiating pain into the shoulders or headaches. •Abdominal pain. •Difficulty swallowing or breathing.

Achenbach's Syndrome:

Described as rare Syndromes, but what if all these Syndromes are only one with many different names? Spontaneous Blue Finger Syndrome, Achenbach's Syndrome (Paroxysmal finger hematoma), or Popped Blood Vessel in Finger. If these Syndromes are all the same, then they are not so uncommon after all.

Achenbach's Syndrome or Paroxysmal Hand Hematoma:

Achenbach syndrome (Paroxysmal finger hematoma) is a rare, benign, and self-limiting condition, which causes bruising, swelling, and burning pain in the hand or fingers. Achenbach's Syndrome appears spontaneously or after a hidden minor trauma and heals completely within days.

Spontaneous Blue Finger Syndrome:

Now, here again, medical reports say that the acute Spontaneous Blue Finger Syndrome is a rare, benign condition, that affects mostly like Achenbach's Syndrome the female population. The finger typically becomes acutely painful and then turns blue and heals completely within days.

Finger Popped Blood Vessel:

Sometimes blood vessels may break for no apparent reason and most often is due to high blood pressure or from a hidden minor trauma.

My Story of Achenbach's Syndrome:
For the first time, my finger hurt in the gym for no apparent reason. I felt only pain but without a bruise. After a week I went shopping and all of a sudden, I felt a sharp pain in my left small finger and within a second it became blue. I immediately panicked, as the first thing that came to my mind was a blood clot. After research, I found out all about the Spontaneous Blue Finger and Achenbach's Syndromes. So, I felt better and now, after 72 hours the bruise is completely gone. I visited a general practitioner just to be sure, and he assured me not to worry because the bruise had already healed.

Rabies Vaccine Side Effects for Humans:

My Personal Experience with Rabies:

So Here I Am, in Pai Thailand, bitten by a dog in a hotel. The boss of the hotel, confirms that his dog had all the necessary vaccines and I shouldn't worry, but I do worry! I immediately went to Pai hospital and the doctor told me that I did the right thing. Even if the bite was not so deep and even if the dog didn't look so dangerous the best thing to do is to visit your nearby clinic or hospital and get an anti-rabies vaccine. So, long story short, the doctor gave me a vaccine shot and told me that I have to do four more. You must visit your doctor five times for full treatment.

Side effects from the vaccine are very common. 5% to 40% of the patients may experience flu-like symptoms, headache, nausea, myalgias, vomiting, upset stomach, or diarrhea. The first shot was fine, but on the second, I had side effects like an upset stomach, dizziness, headache, and more. I'm not sure if it was my GERD or the vaccine. I will be sure when I do the third shot tomorrow. Today I went to all of the clinics here just to check for the right vaccine. When they gave me the first shot in Pai they gave me a vaccine called Abhayram and I didn't have any side effects. The second time they gave me the Verorab vaccine and I had the side effects that I described above. My fear of rabies vaccine side effects makes me look everywhere for Abhayram, but unfortunately, no one has it. So, I have to use Verorab for the second time. The good news is that this time I didn't have any side effects, except a little headache and some dizziness. I'm feeling much better and that is a reliever. I'm sure that the side effects that I had the second time were because of the vaccine, and exercise.

What I did and I had Less Side Effects?

I didn't exercise that day, I ate good and healthy food, I drank a lot of fluids.

Rare Rabies Vaccine Side Effects:

For the first time in my life, I had vertigo a week after the third shot. Vertigo is a scary sensation that the world around you is spinning. I read the causes and one of them was (Certain medications that cause ear damage). I did a research on the internet and I found that there were a few cases of sudden onset unilateral sensorineural hearing loss after rabies vaccination. I don't know if my cause was because of the vaccine or if I had an ear infection or both (I mean the vaccine makes it worst). Sudden hearing loss and neurologic complications including Guillain-Barre syndrome or facial paralysis are reported as side effects after a rabies vaccine.

Conclusions:

Vaccine safety gets more public attention than vaccination. Rabies Vaccine side effects for humans are real but most of the time mild, as modern vaccines get (better).

Change in Guidelines:

The doctors in Thailand told me to do five shots, but because I hate the vaccine toxins I researched and found that CDC guidelines had changed. Now four shots are enough and as a result, we have fewer rabies vaccine side effects.

Rabies vaccine Detoxification:

If you think about it, vaccination is a natural treatment. The only problem is that together with antigens they use some chemicals and other stuff as preservatives and stabilizers for preventing dangerous bacterial and fungal contamination. Immunizations can lead to a negative reaction, mercury, formaldehyde, or aluminum can be toxic to the human body at certain levels.

So how to detox from vaccination?

Consume organic fruits and vegetables because they have detoxifying effects. Fast for a while. Drink pure water. Visit the sauna. Exercise, make use of hot and cold hydrotherapy, and supplement with Activated Charcoal.

The most Important Blood Tests for Men:

Depending on our age, lifestyle factors, and family history, we all need different tests. Men of all ages must do some blood tests to see if they are still healthy, especially Men after 40. That's why I went today to the Medical Laboratory to test myself. We should all visit our health care provider often, even if we feel healthy. A blood test diagnosis has a lot of health benefits as we can avoid problems in the future. So here are the best Lab tests to make.

Diabetes Test:

Here are the most important blood tests for diabetes: The Random blood sugar test, the A1C test (most common test), and the fasting plasma glucose test (FPG) are the best ways to diagnose diabetes.

Sexually Transmitted Infections (STD TEST):

Even if you have a longtime relationship, it's always a good idea to get tested for STDs.

Cholesterol Test:

High cholesterol, usually has no symptoms, and a Cholesterol test is used to predict an individual's risk of developing heart disease! A cholesterol test is called a lipid profile and is measure the good cholesterol (high-density lipoprotein cholesterol – HDL-C) the bad cholesterol (low-density lipoprotein cholesterol – LDL-C) and triglycerides in your blood.

Vitamin D Test:

Vitamin D is not a real vitamin, it's mostly a steroid hormone that you can obtain through sun exposure. It's for sure one of the most important tests for immune function and cancer prevention. The Vitamin D blood test is called a 25(OH)D blood test.

Thyroid Test:

A TSH blood test can check if you have any thyroid gland problems. A lower TSH level could mean that your thyroid it's overactive (hyperthyroidism) and a higher level of TSH could mean that your thyroid is underactive (hypothyroidism).

Other Important Blood Tests for Men:

DHEA Test:

Dehydroepiandrosterone is a hormone produced by the adrenal glands, and is a precursor to testosterone, estrogen, and sex hormones.

Prostate-Specific Antigen Test:

Healthy men have low amounts of PSA in the blood, so Prostate-specific antigen test measures the amount of PSA in the blood. As a result, the test can find if there is inflammation of the prostate gland or prostate cancer.

Iron Test:

Iron is an essential trace element and an iron test is very important. The Serum Iron test is used to evaluate body iron stores or the iron level in blood serum.

Gout Test:

Many guys eat a lot of meat and if you are after 40 is always a good idea to check your uric acid levels. A serum uric acid test can measure how much uric acid is present in your blood.

Top Epidemic-Pandemic Diseases Throughout History:

Ebola Virus:

The Ebola virus was first discovered in 1976 in West Africa. The virus is transmitted among humans through physical contact with infected bodily fluids. Symptoms of Ebola: Aches, headache, joint pain, fatigue, abdominal pain, weakness, diarrhea, and vomiting.

Marburg Virus:

It's a fatal zoonotic disease caused by a virus from the same Ebola virus family. Marburg Virus was first started in 1967 in Europe after importing green monkeys. Symptoms: fever, chills, headache, myalgia, nausea, vomiting, chest pain, weight loss, delirium, shock, sore throat, abdominal pain, and diarrhea.

Bird Flu (Avian Flu):

Bird flu is an influenza virus that mainly affects birds. H5N1 was the first Bird Flu virus (Hong Kong 1997) to infect humans. Avian Flu is transmitted via contact with an infected bird. Bird Flu Symptoms: Diarrhea, cough, headache, runny nose, respiratory difficulties, fever, muscle aches, malaise.

The Black Death:

The Great Plague killed 25 million people across Europe during the mid-14th Century. It is caused by bacteria called Yersinia pestis. We thought that the disease was transmitted by infected fleas living on rats, which would then bite humans. A new study shows evidence that this view is perhaps incorrect.

Instead, human parasites such as fleas and body lice were spreading the plague bacteria during the Second Pandemic. Symptoms: Abdominal pain with diarrhea, weakness, nausea, vomiting, chills, fever, bleeding, and shock.

Plague of Athens:

The Athenian plague of 430 BC – 426 BC killed an estimated 80,000 to 100,000 people. The cause of the plague of Athens continues to be debated. Some experts say that was Measles, Typhoid, or epidemic Typhus, and now some medical studies suggest that was in fact, an attack of Ebola. The Greek physician Hippocrates found the cure for the Plague by burning the infected clothes and by bringing fresh drinking water from Kos Island. Symptoms: High fever, weakness, muscle pain, chills, diarrhea, headache, lack of appetite.

Smallpox:

Today we speak about smallpox like it's not a big deal, but once was one of the world's most feared diseases. The first Smallpox vaccine was discovered in the late 1700s. Smallpox's earliest evidence was found in Egypt 3,000 years ago but it's believed to have appeared around 10,000 BC. 300 million people died from smallpox in the 20th century alone. Smallpox Symptoms: Sudden onset of high fever, diarrhea, skin rash with flat spots/raised bumps, headache, backache, and abdominal pain with vomiting.

Measles:

Measles Virus (Rubeola) lives within the mucus of the patient nose and throat and it is spread through the air with direct contact same as the common flu. A new study show evidence that it appeared about 4,000 years ago. Before the vaccine, Measles epidemics affected millions every year. In the 60s, measles infected about 4 million people in the United States. Measles Symptoms: Runny nose, sneezing, swollen-watery eyes, white spots in the mouth, red eyes, high-temperature fever aches, and pains.

Tuberculosis:

The bacteria Mycobacterium tuberculosis is highly contagious and was the world's deadliest. It's still the number one cause of death among infectious diseases globally. TB epidemic in Europe and North America killed one out of every seven people during the 18th and 19th centuries. The BCG (Bacille Calmette-Guérin) vaccine was discovered in 1921. Tuberculosis Symptoms: Cough, chest pain, night sweats, coughing up blood, fever, weakness, chills, loss of appetite.

Malaria:

Malaria is a prehistoric origin, a zoonotic disease caused by infection of Plasmodium protozoa, transmitted by an infective female Anopheles mosquito. This disease first travels to a human's liver, grows, and then travels into the bloodstream and destroys the red blood cells. Malaria kills about 2 million people every year, and 90% of the deaths are located in Africa. Malaria Symptoms: Chills, high fever, headache, nausea, sweating, vomiting, diarrhea, and abdominal pain.

The Plague of Justinian:

The Justinianic Plague was a pandemic disease that exterminates Constantinople and the entire Byzantine Empire. In 541 CE, the Plague of Justinian infected millions in just a year. It is estimated to have killed between 30 and 50 million people. The disease took its name from the Byzantine emperor at the time Justinian. Symptoms of the Justinianic Plague: fever, chills, headache, swollen lymph nodes, abdominal pain, and delusions.

The Spanish Flu:

One of the deadliest diseases in history was the Spanish flu pandemic of 1918. Infected an estimated one-third of the planet's population and killed about 30 million people. Symptoms of Spanish Flu: Nausea, aches, diarrhea, headache, chills, sweats, cough, weakness, vomiting, sore throat.

The Antonine Plague:

Another ancient pandemic. The Antonine Plague of the Roman Empire flared up during the time of Marcus Aurelius in 165 AD. The famous Greek physician Galen found himself in the middle of this pandemic. This disease nearly broke the Roman Empire apart and killed around five million people. Symptoms of the Antonine Plague: Diarrhea, fever, pharyngitis, and rashes.

Typhus:

Epidemic Typhus is a bacterial disease caused by Rickettsia Prowazekii, it first appeared in 1489. Spread to humans by animals-fleas such as cats, rats, raccoons, and so on... Typhus Symptoms: fever, high fever, nausea, vomiting, diarrhea, delirium, headache, and rash.

Asian Flu:
The Asian flu pandemic of 1956 (H2N2 virus), killed around one million to two million people worldwide. Lasted until 1958 and was one of the most famous influenza pandemics in history. Fortunately, a vaccine against the H2N2 virus and antibiotics limited the spread of the pandemic. Asian Flu Symptoms: Cough, fever, body aches, chills, weakness, loss of appetite.

Pertussis:
Pertussis is a highly contagious respiratory tract infection disease known as whooping cough and is caused by a type of bacteria called Bordetella pertussis. Whooping cough is a very serious respiratory infection but can be treated with antibiotics. Various epidemics have been described from 1906 until now. The bacteria Bordetella pertussis spreads from person to person in airborne droplets or with direct contact. Pertussis symptoms: Low-grade fever, runny nose, weakness, mild cough.

Leprosy (Hansen's disease):
Leprosy grew into a pandemic in the medieval period of European history. Was believed to be a punishment from God like a karma disease. Today can be treated with antibiotics. Leprosy Symptoms: Skin sores, muscle weakness, skin lumps and bumps, loss of sensation, skin ulcers, numbness in the hands, legs, arms, feet.

Cholera:

Cholera is an ancient problem caused by a bacterium called Vibrio Cholerae. In 1817, cholera caused a very lethal outbreak in India and spread to other countries in Asia. Since then, we had seven global pandemics of cholera worldwide. Cholera Symptoms: Diarrhea and watery stools, dehydration, low blood pressure, vomiting, dry mouth, rapid heart rate.

Polio:

Poliomyelitis is a highly contagious infectious disease, caused by a virus (poliovirus) that can lead to paralysis. Polio is an ancient disease but polio epidemics started for the first time in the 19th century. Poliomyelitis can strike people at any age and around 95 percent of all cases are asymptomatic. Polio Symptoms: fever, muscle weakness, back and neck pain, nausea, sore throat, headache, vomiting, joint pain, fatigue.

HIV/AIDS:

HIV/AIDS is a sexually transmitted infection spread with certain body fluids like blood, semen, pre-seminal fluid, vaginal fluids, rectal fluids, and breast milk. Scientific data suggests that the AIDS epidemic started in the late 1970s and 1980 HIV has already spread Globally. HIV destroys some white blood cells of the immune system, called CD4 cells. AIDS is the most advanced stage of HIV infection. Today, the Human immunodeficiency virus has become a manageable chronic health condition. HIV/AIDS Symptoms: rapid weight loss, fever, chronic fatigue, diarrhea, unexplained tiredness, swelling of the lymph glands, chills and night sweats, rashes, sores of the mouth, anus, and genitals, pneumonia.

Hong Kong flu 1968:

The Hong Kong flu pandemic of 1968 was highly contagious and caused by an H3N2 strain of the influenza A virus. This virus killed over a million lives worldwide, with most excess deaths in people 65 years and older. Hong Kong flu Symptoms: Fever, chills, weakness, and muscle pain.

Russian Flu 1889:

The 1889 pandemic, began in Russia and spread rapidly throughout Europe and the world. Russian Flu (H1N1) killed around 1 million people. The virus was first recorded in Saint Petersburg. Russian Flu Symptoms: Fever, fatigue, chills, cough, and body aches.

Should I Remove Clavicle Plates?

Many patients who have titanium plates ask the same question: Do I need to remove the titanium plates after surgery? I had a very bad motorcycle accident n my early 20s. My leg broke and the doctors added a titanium plate to my left leg. I had very bad luck as after the operation I got an infection from the surgical wound. So, they had to put me in the operating room for a second time. For all these reasons I was afraid of removing the osteosynthesis materials. The materials had to be removed as soon as the fracture healed. Until now, I wasn't sure if I was doing the right thing, and holding the titanium plate in my foot for so long. I did some research. Many surgeons recommend leaving surgical titanium plates in unless a patient requests to take them out. Unfortunately, complications can occur after the material is removed. Patients generally want to remove the material only if it causes discomfort. In children and teenagers, it is usually recommended to remove the metalware and clavicle plates early to avoid disturbances to the growing skeleton. Unfortunately, complications can occur when doctors remove the hardware. As an example: Nearby nerves can be injured during the process. In my case, my left leg is a point shorter than the right one and as a result, I get problems after a workout. Problems like mild paresthesias in my extremes. The good news is that the more I exercise the stronger I get.

Lump in the Throat Causes:

Some people experience an odd sensation of having something stuck in their throat 10 to 20 minutes after eating. What may cause it? The feeling of something stuck at the back of the throat can be caused by many causes. The lump in the throat sensation is also called Gobus Pharyngeus. People with Gobus Pharyngeus usually don't have a problem when eating or drinking and this weird sensation tends to come and go. There are many theories of what can cause the lump in the throat sensation, but some specialists believe that the main problem is with the coordination of swallowing muscles. Acid reflux is one of the most serious reasons, as stomach acid affects the relaxation of the muscles around the throating.

Laryngitis:

The larynx is also known as the voice box and is an organ in the neck of tetrapods that is involved in breathing.

Pharyngitis:

Inflammation of the pharynx is caused by viruses or bacteria.

Cricopharyngeal Spasm:

These spasms are usually harmless and occur in the cricopharyngeus muscle of the pharynx. Gastroesophageal Reflux (GERD) and Laryngopharyngeal reflux (LPR): Gastroesophageal Reflux is a digestive disorder that affects the lower esophageal sphincter. During the LPR condition acid made in the stomach travels up the esophagus (swallowing tube).

Allergies and Food Allergies:

Food allergy can irritate and swell the throat. People with allergies, chronic rhinitis, and sinusitis can have a post-nasal drip that can cause a Globus sensation at the back of the throat.

Thyroid disorders:

An underactive thyroid gland can cause a sensation of a lump in the throat.

Emotional Stress:

Emotional stress and anxiety can also cause the Globus sensation.

Lump Behind Ear Lobe Causes:

I know it's scary to have bumps or lumps on your skin. I was scared ten years ago when I saw a small lump behind my ear lobe! That's why I made some research about it and I can tell you that is nothing to worry about, as most of the time is a result of different infections like mastoiditis or even an allergic reaction. Lumps found behind the ear can be small, large, painful, or painless. In most cases, nodules behind the ears are harmless.

Lump Behind Ear Lobe Causes:

Abscess:

An abscess is when your body responds to the infection by trying to kill the invading bacteria or virus.

Acne Vulgaris:

A common skin condition that occurs when hair follicles in the skin become clogged.

Mastoiditis and Otitis Media:

Mastoiditis is an ear infection that could spread to the mastoid bone at the back of your ear. Ear infections can be bacterial or viral.

Dermatitis:

Dermatitis is a general term that describes an inflammation of the skin.

Swollen Lymph Nodes:

Your lymph nodes belong to your immune system and fight infections! A lump behind the ear most usually results from a swollen lymph node, from common infections such as tonsillitis, colds, and flu.

Sebaceous Cysts:

Sebaceous cysts form just under the skin and may be felt like a lump behind the ear. They are less dangerous and often disappear with time.

Throat Infection:

A throat infection can cause swelling in and around your neck. Sinusitis, Allergies, and LPR can cause a Throat infection.

Lipoma:

A lipoma is a slow growth of a fatty lump that is usually found just below the skin!

The Strangest Medical Conditions and Syndromes:

When you watch medical shows like House, The Resident, New Amsterdam, and others, you learn a lot about healthcare, medical diagnosis, rare diseases, and syndromes. Here I've compiled a list of some of the strangest medical conditions and syndromes.

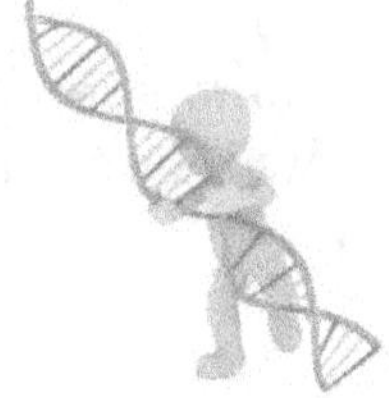

Cysticercosis: Cysticercosis is a parasitic tissue infection caused by larval cysts of the tapeworm Taenia solium.

Psittacosis: An infectious disease usually spread to humans from infected birds in the parrot family.

Osteomyelitis: Osteomyelitis is an infection in a bone. It is usually caused by bacteria or fungi.

Couvade Syndrome: Couvade syndrome happens when a pregnant woman's partner has symptoms that uncannily mimic pregnancy.

Brucellosis: Brucellosis is an infectious disease caused by bacteria.

Tick Borne Disease: Lyme disease is transmitted by the blacklegged tick (bacterium Borrelia burgdorferi and rarely, Borrelia mayonii).

Naegleria Fowleri: Naegleria Fowleri infects people when water contains the ameba and enters the body through the nose and travels to the brain, where it destroys brain tissue.

Addison's Disease: Addison's disease is an uncommon disorder that occurs when your body doesn't produce enough of certain hormones.

Eyes Parasites and Worms List: Onchocerca volvulus, Acanthamoeba castellanii, Toxocara cati - Toxocara canis, Thelazia callipaeda, baylisascaris procyonis, nematodes, cestodes - trematodes ascariasis worm, Loa Loa Worm.

Chronic Granulomatous Disease: CGD is a genetic disorder in which white blood cells called phagocytes are unable to kill certain types of bacteria and fungi.

Erythropoietic Protoporphyria: EPP is a rare inherited metabolic disorder caused by a deficiency of the enzyme ferrochelatase (FECH).

Congenital Insensitivity Disease: CIPA is a rare autosomal recessive disorder of the nervous system which prevents the feeling of pain.

Human Tapeworm: The tapeworm is a parasite that lives in the gut. Eating undercooked meat from infected animals is the main cause of tapeworm infection.

Mass Psychogenic Illness: MPI happens when people in a group start feeling sick at the same time even though there is no physical reason for them to be sick.

Hemochromatosis: Hemochromatosis is a disorder in which extra iron builds up in the body to harmful levels.

Synesthesia: Synesthesia in Greek is "to perceive together" and is an anomalous blending of the senses, for example, people hear a word and instantly see a color.

Fat Embolism: Fat embolism syndrome occurs when fat enters the bloodstream.

Chagas Disease: This is a tropical parasitic disease caused by Trypanosoma cruzi.

Gastric Trichobezoar: A trichobezoar is a mass of undigested hair within the gastrointestinal tract.

Lucio Phenomenon: LP is a rare reactional state seen in cases of diffuse lepromatous leprosy.

Sjogren's Syndrome: Sjogren's syndrome is a disorder of the immune system and has symptoms like dry eyes and a dry mouth.

Familial Mediterranean Fever: FMF is a genetic autoinflammatory disorder that causes recurrent fevers and painful inflammation.

Melioidosis: Whitmore's disease is an infectious disease caused by the bacterium Burkholderia pseudomallei.

Hereditary Coproporphyria: Hereditary coproporphyria is a rare metabolic disorder characterized by a deficiency of the enzyme coproporphyrinogen oxidase.

Parthenogenesis in Humans: Parthenogenesis is the development of an unfertilized female sex cell without any male contribution.

Doege Potter Syndrome: This is a rare paraneoplastic syndrome that is often diagnosed incidentally during the workup of hypoglycemia of unclear etiology.

Sporotrichosis in Humans: This cutaneous skin infection, occurs when a fungus enters the skin through a small cut after someone touches contaminated plant matter.

Intracranial Berry Aneurysm: Brain aneurysms can occur in any blood vessel that supplies the brain.

Vibrio Vulnificus: Vibrio vulnificus is a marine bacterial infection and is the leading cause of death related to seafood consumption in the United States.

Hughes Stovin Syndrome: HSS is a rare autoimmune disorder, characterized by deep venous thrombosis and bronchial aneurysms.

Whipple's Disease: Whipple disease is a rare bacterial infection that affects joints and the digestive system.

Henoch-schonlein Purpura: HSP is a disease involving inflammation of small blood vessels and most commonly occurs in children.

Rickettsialpox: Rickettsialpox is a mild disease caused by the bacterial organism Rickettsia akari.

Cobalt Poisoning: Cobalt poisoning is an intoxication caused by excessive levels of cobalt in the body.

Mcleod Syndrome: This syndrome is primarily a neurological disorder that occurs almost exclusively in boys and men.

Muckle Wells Disease: MWS is a rare genetic autoinflammatory syndrome.

Refsum Disease: It's an inherited condition that causes vision loss, anosmia, and many other symptoms.

Ehlers-Danlos Syndrome: EDS is a group of inherited disorders that affect your connective tissues.

Mastocytosis: Mastocytosis is a rare condition caused by an excess number of mast cells gathering in the body's tissues.

Plummer's Disease: This thyroid condition is characterized by marked enlargement of the thyroid gland (goitre).

Jarisch Herxheimer Reaction: JHR is a reaction to endotoxin-like products released by the death of harmful microorganisms within the body during antibiotic treatment.

Rare Alport Syndrome: Another rare genetic disorder characterized by progressive kidney disease and abnormalities of the inner ear and the eye.

Amoebiasis: This is a condition in which your gut becomes infected with the parasite E. histolytica.

Diphtheria: Diphtheria is a serious infection caused by strains of bacteria called Corynebacterium diphtheriae that make toxins.

Cellular Memory: CM is the hypothesis that (traumatic) memories can be stored in individual cells outside the brain.

Wegener's Granulomatosis: Granulomatosis with polyangiitis (formerly called Wegener's) is a rare disease.

Measles: Measles can result in 'immune amnesia.' Children infected with measles must be vaccinated again for diseases against which they have previously been immunized.

Auto Brewery Syndrome: This condition happens when ethanol is produced through endogenous fermentation by fungi or bacteria in the gastrointestinal system.

Teratomas: Teratomas are a rare type of tumor born from genetic anomalies and reproduce organs (hair, muscle, teeth, and bone). Some teratomas create antibodies that attack the brain and lead to encephalitis.

Cryptococcosis Fungal Infection: This fungus infection may be spread to humans through contact with pigeon droppings or unwashed raw fruit.

Polyarteritis Nodosa: PAN is a rare disease that results from blood vessel inflammation-causing injury to organ systems.

Porphyria: A group of disorders that result from a buildup of natural chemicals that produce porphyrin in your body.

Androgen Insensitivity Syndrome: AIS occurs when someone is genetically male but is resistant to male sex hormones.

Pheochromocytoma: A pheochromocytoma is a rare, usually non-cancerous tumor that develops in an adrenal gland.

Pulmonary Alveolar Proteinosis: PAP is a set of symptoms and signs, a rare lung disease caused by a build-up of material in the air sacs.

Palinopsia: Palinopsia is rare, it is caused by HPPD, migraines, prescription drugs, or head trauma. In Greek means again seeing, (Palin = again and opsia = seeing).

Ehlers Danlos Syndrome: EDS is a group of rare inherited conditions that affect connective tissues supporting the skin, bones, blood vessels, and many other organs and tissues.

Chiari malformation: Chiari malformation is a condition in which brain tissue extends into the spinal canal. Type III is extremely rare.

Moyamoya: Moyamoya is a chronic, rare and progressive condition of the arteries in the brain.

Genetic Mitochondrial Disease: Mitochondrial diseases are individually uncommon, but collectively pose a significant burden on human health.

Rapunzel Syndrome: This syndrome is an extremely rare condition with an unusual form of trichobezoar that is seen in patients with a history of psychiatric disorders.

Acute Compartment Syndrome: ACS is a medical emergency, usually caused by trauma.

Positive and Negative Effects of Masturbation:

Today, it is considered safe, but masturbation has not always been socially acceptable and refers more to men than women. Many believe that masturbation can quickly become an addiction and they are right. There is no such thing as the ideal number to masturbate as the frequency depends on a person's age, lifestyle, and overall health. Masturbation has positive and negative effects and that's the reason that should be done moderately.

Here are Some Positive Effects of Masturbation:
It helps you sleep. It's a Muscle relaxant, stress-reducer, and mood-enhancer. It prevents prostate cancer and alleviates urinary tract infections.

Here are Some Negatives Effects:
Masturbation and our immune system: While this habit is known to be fun for some, it can be an activity that affects negatively our immune system. When an individual masturbates too often, his body loses some necessary chemicals. Weakness, frequent urination, and loss of immunity in the whole body are very common problems in individuals with the habit of masturbation. Unfortunately, it's also the main cause of erectile dysfunction. Masturbation stressors in a person's emotions can cause sexual dysfunction. Strain in a relationship: Your partner may think she/he is not enough for you. This habit makes you lonely. People who masturbate too often will lose interest in sex.

Phantosmia Causes:

Phantosmia is the phenomenon of smelling things that simply aren't there (phantom smell). It is also known as an "olfactory hallucination". The smell of Phantosmia disorder is usually unpleasant (Smoke, Gas, Ammonia) and can spoil your taste. If you write phantosmia causes in almost every search engine out there, the worst cases (like always) are at the top of the search results and this is not accidental. Fear is the best way to give anxiety to people. Just remember, most phantom smells go away in time and are not caused by something serious. The first thing you have to do is to be sure that the smell is not there, because sometimes we all confuse things.

Phantosmia Causes:

Aging. Drugs. Sinusitis. Allergies. Nasal surgery. Dental problems. Hypothyroidism. Smoking. Exposure to certain chemicals. Migraine with aura. COVID.

Antibiotic Resistance in Gonorrhea:

Gonorrhea is a sexually transmitted disease and has existed since medieval times. Is an infection caused by the bacteria Neisseria gonorrhea and can affect your urethra, rectum, throat, or eyes! People with gonorrhea have symptoms like Pain (burning) in Urethra, swelling of the testicles, vaginal discharge, and anal itching. Gonorrhea used to be known as "the clap".

Gonorrhea While Using a Condom:

Unfortunately, gonorrhea is easily passed between people, even with oral sex or even if they use a condom. Condoms can reduce the risk of contracting sexually transmitted diseases but not 100 percent. Touching infected sex organs, and then touching yours it's enough to get an infection.

Symptoms for Males:

Pain when peeing. Need to pee more often. Unusual fluid from the penis. An itchy feeling inside the penis. Swelling in the testicles. Anal itching.

Symptoms for Females:

More painful periods. Vaginal bleeding after sex. Pain in the lower stomach. Painful or frequent urination. Anal itching. General tiredness.

Antibiotic Resistance in Gonorrhea:

It used to be easy to cure gonorrhea with antibiotics, but gonorrhea has developed resistance to many antibiotic drugs prescribed to treat it. That means that today's gonorrhea patient has very few treatment options left. Some experts even say that soon Gonorrhea is about to become impossible to treat. Today, Dr. Kevin Fenton, former director of the CDC's agency on sexually transmitted diseases, advises treating gonorrhea with an injectable drug called ceftriaxone.

Why are People Feeling Sick After Shower?

Do you feel sick after taking a shower? Are your daily showers bad for your health? It is very common. Let's look at the reasons, and why are people feeling sick after a shower. First, hot water can raise your blood pressure and hyper-stimulate the immune system which can make you experience flu-like symptoms like light-headed, runny or stuffy nose, nausea, sneezing, chills, fatigue, or dyspnea. But what about cold water? Probably the immune system gets weak, because of the addition of chemicals in public water like Chlorine. Chlorine is a chemical typically used as a disinfectant, to reduce the level of pathogenic bacteria in our drinking water. You ingest more chemicals from one shower through your skin and from breathing in the steam than you do from drinking water all day. In people with weak immune systems and allergies, those chemicals inside the water can make you feel sick. Another serious reason is dehydration. If you are not drinking enough fluids, you could be dehydrated and get all of those symptoms.

Solution:

Reverse dehydration by drinking more fluids. Try to take shorter showers and run the cold water for the last few minutes so it can help counter all of these symptoms.

Is Fluoride Good or Bad for our Health?

Fluoride is an inorganic anion that occurs naturally in many foods and water. Most people are exposed to fluorides daily. CDC claims that water fluoridation is one of the greatest health achievements of the 20th century. But, it's fluoride good or bad for our health? Some people think fluoride in drinking water is a good thing and some say just the opposite! Many things can be good for you in moderation, but seriously harmful in large amounts. On the other hand, some people are allergic or sensitive to fluoride. People with allergies to fluoride need to be more careful about brushing their teeth. There are two main forms of fluoride. The natural version is known as calcium fluoride and is not so harmful. Now, the synthetic industrial version is called sodium fluoride and can be harmful. Also, Fluoridation is not a "Natural" process. Most developed countries do not fluoridate their water.

Natural Glutamic Acid vs Manufactured:

Glutamic acid is produced inside the human body. For humans, it is a non-essential amino acid. Glutamic acid also occurs naturally in many foods such as parmesan cheese, mushrooms, and soybean products. Glutamates that occur naturally in food contain different chemicals and fiber, which the body is naturally inclined to regulate. MSG glutamic acid is produced outside the human body and not naturally like in the foods above. Everything started when the Japanese scientist Kikunae Ikeda, was able to isolate the main substance of dashi–the seaweed Laminaria japonica. Now instead of four tastes: sweet, salty, bitter, and sour, we have five. He called this new taste, umami, from the Japanese Umai (delicious). Most people don't know that umami and MSG is the same thing. The short answer is that MSG is synthetic glutamate and most of the time is accompanied by impurities. It is produced from both wheat gluten and sugar beet molasses.

Wheat-derived MSG has been found in products imported from Asia. MSG is connected with subsequent learning, brain damage, and endocrine disorders. MSG causes reactions in many people such as •Headaches. •Tingling in the mouth •Sleepiness •Shortness of breath •Nausea. •Numbness •Skin rash •Heart palpitations. •Lightheadedness. •Ringing Ears.

Tinnitus and Fleeting Tinnitus Causes:

Tinnitus is very common, about 1 in 100 people have problems with tinnitus which affects their quality of life. Most of us will experience this ringing of sounds in the ears at some time, but tinnitus can be extremely disturbing to people who have it, especially those who have chronic tinnitus. The sort of noises that people hear includes ringing, clicking, buzzing, whooshing, whistles, roaring, hissing, crickets, pulsing, screeching, sirens, static, ocean waves, buzzing, humming, machine type noises, etc. Fleeting When you have tinnitus, your hearing is reduced and you hear a loud, high-pitched ringing in one or both of your ears. Most of the time it just happens out of the blue but is a little frightening when it happens. Many people that experienced fleeting tinnitus often panic, but just relax and it will soon go away. In some cases, tinnitus is related to another problem. I do not experience fleeting tinnitus often, but when happens it is because of my neck pain or my allergies and sinusitis problems. Fleeting Tinnitus is temporary tinnitus. Tinnitus is just a symptom and does not cause hearing loss.

Causes:

Exposure to loud noise. Sinusitis or allergies. Earwax blockage. Ear bone changes. Meniere's disease. Head or neck injuries. Inner ear damage. Middle ear infection. Anemia. Acoustic neuroma. Some Medications.

Hidden Inflammation the Chronic Enemy:

Inflammation activates chemicals in the body after the reactive effect on various harmful factors such as bacteria, viruses, chemicals, injuries, etc. The infections are divided into acute (lasting a few days) and chronic (longer). Cells play an important role in the mechanism of inflammation, such as macrophages and leukocytes, which are arriving at the site of inflammation through blood circulation. Consequences of this inflammatory process are some clinical phenomena that are characteristic of inflammation. These phenomena are Pain, Edema (swelling), redness, and heat. Inflammation has been recognized as the substrate for almost every chronic disease. Diseases like asthma, rheumatoid arthritis, Crohn's disease, diabetes, depression, Alzheimer's disease, and heart disease. In recent years we have evidence showing that chronic inflammation may be implicated in the transition from the precancerous stage to the stage of a full disease.

Foods that Cause Chronic Inflammation:

New research linking lifestyle and diet with inflammation and susceptibility to disease. Obesity, heart disease, cancer, osteoporosis, and depression are associated with what we eat. The foods that promote inflammation include processed foods that provide many calories and have lost most of their nutritional value. Such foods are sugar, white flour, and high-sodium processed foods. These foods when entering the body affect insulin and blood sugar levels. The sugar initially rises sharply and then falls abruptly. This causes increased hormone secretions that create inflammation. Our body in its effort to keep the blood sugar to desired levels increases insulin secretion. Elevated levels of insulin in the blood have been correlated with increased levels of inflammatory.

Anti-Inflammatory Foods:

If we eat foods that promote chronic diseases, even if the sugar levels in our blood are in the normal range, we may have elevated insulin levels and a predisposition to inflammation. Eating foods with a low glycemic index is beneficial to our health and has anti-inflammatory properties. Such foods are green vegetables, olive oil, organic eggs, and barley rusks. Raw foods are rich in nutrients and have a low glycemic index. Such foods are raw nuts, seeds, fruits, and berries. Organic foods that contain natural vitamins, minerals, protein, and enzymes provide our body with the essential raw materials and ensure good health.

Hidden Inflammation Symptoms and Signs:

Hidden chronic inflammation is not perceived because it causes no pain. As a result, the patient does nothing to stop the spread of hidden inflammation. The inflammation hides for years, if not decades, and is perceived only when eventually causes damage to the organs. How can you know if you are suffering from hidden inflammation and what to do to treat it? These questions can show you if something is wrong with your body: Are you suffering from obesity? Do you use antidepressants? Do you use cholesterol medications? Are you suffering from chronic fatigue? Are you suffering from a lack of concentration? Do you desire sugar and starch? Do you suffer from constipation? Are you suffering from insomnia? Do you suffer from headaches? Are you suffering from dry skin? Do you suffer from regular colds? Are you feeling exhausted, especially after exercise? Are you feeling unwell and you don't know the reason? If you answer yes to more than three questions, then you have elevated levels of hidden chronic inflammation. No drug can reverse the high levels of hidden inflammation. The anti-inflammatory zone diet accomplishes. It has been clinically proven, that within 30 days, there is a significant reduction of the hidden inflammation. Control your diet to maintain wellness throughout your life. When you consume foods that are closer to their natural state and strengthen the antioxidant mechanisms in your body, the inflammation is reduced.

Itchy Skin After Swimming in a Pool:

Today I visited a friend's hotel swimming pool. When I got out of the pool, my skin was extremely dry, and after about twenty minutes, I noticed that it was burning and itching. Chlorine is a common problem for those who swim in swimming pools. Chlorine is a cleaning agent in swimming pools to prevent bacterial growth. Itchy is an irritating sensation that makes you want to scratch. Serious itching can be caused by allergies and infections. Chlorine is corrosive and can cause allergies and sensitivities (chlorine sensitivity or chlorine allergy). Sometimes those irritations are happening only because of the dryness of the skin. Itching skin can affect a small area of the skin or the full body. Chlorine in the swimming pool causes our skin to become dry and itchy, but you don't have to give up swimming. What you might do is use a swimming pool that has the correct chlorine levels. Shower immediately before and after swimming in the pool. Pools with saltwater are preferred. Put on a protective cream when staying in the sun, and don't stay in the sunlight too long.

Number of Bacteria in Human Body:

Have you ever wondered if you are the only creature that lives in your body? Sometimes ignorance is bliss. It's not easy accepting the fact that billions of other organisms live with us. The Human body is a microcosm of the environment around us. Did you know that our hair is just dead cells? The number of bacteria outnumbers human cells by a ratio of at least 10:1 in the human body. According to recent research by the National Institutes of Health (NIH), 90% of cells in the human body are bacterial, fungal, or in other words, non-human organisms. Most of these microscopic hitchhikers are harmless, and some are crucial for a healthy life. With the help of technology and some special micro-cameras, scientists recorded both the bacteria that live in our bodies, but also their various microorganisms that are one trillion times smaller than the head of a pin. That is an unknown microcosm that sometimes scares us. Is our body a caterpillar and our soul the butterfly? I hope so, One thing is certain: most of the microorganisms that live inside our bodies serve a purpose!

Post Flu Symptoms and Flu Complications:

Rebuild your body after the flu is not always an easy project. Normally, symptoms of flu start after two to three days and a person begins to feel better within five to nine days. Some people have a strong immune system and some do not. That's why the flu can affect people in different ways. However, some post-flu symptoms like a lingering cough or feeling tired for two to three weeks after are considered normal. Some of the flu complications may be mild, while others can be life-threatening. Flu complications such as sinusitis (sinus infections), ear infections, asthma, bronchitis, or even pneumonia are examples of bad complications from flu. The flu can make chronic health problems also to get worse. Some people may have cough stick around for a long time. This post-flu cough happens because the virus attacks lung tissue (cilia) and causes irritation. That happened to me once, after a strong virus infection. I had fatigue, nausea, sore throat, stuffy nose, and phlegm for two weeks after the infection. So if you have had post-flu symptoms for more than a month contact your doctor for a follow-up exam.

Some Medical Conspiracy
Theories are Real:

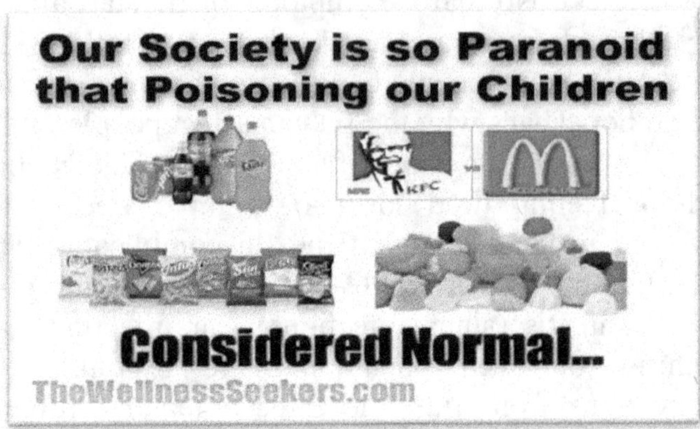

A common misconception is that all people that believe in conspiracy theories and supernatural phenomena are grounded in illusory pattern perception. Some experts believe that conspiracy theorists are easily fooled by things that may not exist, this phenomenon is referred to in psychology as an illusory pattern. While that theory may be true in some cases in many others is wrong, as many of these conspiracy theories proved to be true. We already know many US national security conspiracy theories that turned out to be legit. Or, real conspiracy theories about health like "The Project Sunshine", "The Bad booze", "The LSD Government mind control", "The Dental Amalgam Toxicity" (that was called conspiracy theory and today it's called dental amalgam controversy or dilemma) and "The Operation Berkshire".

Tobacco companies used doctors for decades to promote cigarettes and buried evidence that smoking is deadly and causes lung cancer, heart disease, emphysema, and other serious diseases. R.J. Reynolds Tobacco Company launched an ad campaign with the slogan, "More doctors smoke Camels than any other cigarette." In 1946 another campaign was. "DDT so safe you can eat it" In 1947, some Governments including the USA, sprayed DDT (dichloro-diphenyl-trichloroethane) on people and even children in Texas. But what about the conspiracy theories of our time? Do we have any evidence that proves that any of these medical conspiracy theories are real? I made some research and I have found that some of these conspiracy theories are maybe real.

Codex Alimentarius Conspiracy:

Does the big pharma want to control health supplements? No one will be able to buy or sell food if not approved by the global organization. Codex Alimentarius is one of the major bodies behind the effort to limit access to nutritional products and information. Have you ever heard of Codex Alimentarius? Some say that this evil agenda, which was for long a secret in closed boardrooms and governmental chambers, is now come to light.

What is Codex Alimentarius?

In 1963, the United Nations created a world trade commission to control the world's food supply. The UN calls this code, Codex Alimentarius. Behind the Codex Alimentarius is the United Nations and the World Health Organization. Membership in Codex is open to all member nations of the United Nations (UN) and currently, 165 countries participate. We already not be able to own livestock or any other farm animal without obtaining government permission. They plan to eradicate organic farming & destroy the Natural Health Industry. We found a lot of evidence that many health problems are caused by the use of GMOs (Genetically Modified Organisms). Several animal studies indicate serious health risks associated with genetically modified. Monsanto is the world's leading producer of the world's genetically modified GMO seeds. Although these seeds have been found to cause long-term harmful side effects to animals and humans, the U.N. has for many years now protected these GMO seeds and promoted them worldwide.

The Bayer-Monsanto Conspiracy:

Monsanto approved the bid of $ 66 billion by Bayer. An evil marriage just started. Bayer and Monsanto decided to work together and rule the world by copying and reproducing nature. That is possible only through the Law of Patent worldwide. Monsanto is against natural fertilizers. That means that you are not allowed to irrigate and cherish the plants of your gardens with natural substances. But pesticides are allowed and according to Codex Alimentarius, natural and homemade fertilizers gradually will be prohibited.

The History of Bayer:

Today is one of the biggest pharmaceutical companies in the world. Mostly famous for inventing aspirin, but the dirty history of Bayer is long. During World War, I and II Bayer was a key manufacturer of munitions and explosives for the German government, (TNT), mustard gas, military-grade chlorine, and phosgene. Bayer was then a subsidiary of IG Farben, one of the many pharmaceutical companies connected with the Nazi leadership. Among others, Bayer bought prisoners in WWII to experiment with them. Bayer also invented Heroin, which supposedly made the soldiers 'heroic'.

Bayer and HIV Vaccines:

Unfortunately, is not a hoax and not a conspiracy theory, it is just a conspiracy! According to many websites and news channels, Bayer paid millions of dollars to end a three-decade-long scandal in which the company sold HIV-contaminated blood products to hemophiliacs that were then contaminated with HIV due to the vaccine.

Bayer and the Honeybee Crisis:

Bayer is the exclusive patent holder of imidacloprid, synthetic nicotine, which is most commonly known as Merit and causes CCD, (Colony Collapse Disorder). Colony collapse disorder is a strange phenomenon. All the worker bees of the colony disappear and leave behind the queen together with the immature bees and a few nurse bees, so they can take care of them. Bayer is acting also as a corporate bully, trying to silence campaigners who are standing up for bees".

Subliminal Messages and how Affect our Health:
This theory is about the subliminal messages and how are altering our subconscious and health. Is it true, that there is an elite group of people that control this world? Who are they? The subliminal messages are everywhere in music, movies, video games, etc., and hide a lot of health dangers. Subliminal messages are messages sent directly to the impressionable subconscious mind. Images popped up on movie screens since 1957, but the problem is that people don't see everything that is on the screens, at least not consciously. Companies use these kinds of messages to persuade customers to act in certain ways, but is it a message you want to receive? Our subconscious mind is very powerful and everything we think and believe is stored there. So, in one way, these companies are building characters. How dangerous is that? Subliminal messages are so dangerous that the U.S. Government tried to Ban them from TV and radio back in the '70s. Many people believe that this elite group is a made-up conspiracy theory, and many others believe that exist and started in the 18th century! The Illuminati are maybe a secret society that has been around since 1776, (although the real story goes more back to the times of knights of Templars). It was founded by a Bavarian Professor of Law, a man named Adam Weishaupt. Illuminati wants to create one world government so they can control and manipulate humans. Some people think Illuminati is fake, but the Elite who wants to enslave humanity is real! One of the globalist's favorite tactics is to leave blueprints of their plans with signs "hidden in plain view." From messages delivered to the masses through the media and films.

Denver Airport and Subliminal Messages:

Denver International Airport seems like any other modern airport, but it is not. There are a decent number of conspiracies surrounding the Denver International Airport. Many people believe that the Denver International airport was designed and built by the Elites. The occult concept of "hidden in plain sight" is evidenced by the disturbing symbols used in the murals. An aerial view of the Denver International airport shows that the airport looks like a swastika! One of the strangest things is that Queen Elizabeth II and other important world diplomats have purchased property near the airport. What's up with the creepy apocalyptic paintings in Denver International Airport? Many conspiracy researchers tried to explain the secret meanings of the murals and symbolism around the airport!

Subliminal Messages in Games:

There are many games and video games that predicted the future and the Illuminati card game is one of them. The Illuminati game is a standalone card game made in 1995 by Steve Jackson Games! Steve Jackson Games is a game company founded in 1980 by Steve Jackson. The game is about ominous secret societies competing with each other to control the world. What is strange is that while Steve Jackson was planning to create his first game (Illuminati game) the secret service of the USA raided his office and confiscated his computer equipment. This game has indeed cards that predict the future since 1994.

The Chemtrails Conspiracy:

I never took seriously the Chemtrails conspiracy until I saw the documentary "Why in the World are They Spraying?" Some people think that the trails we see behind airplanes, are not a condensation of water vapor from the hot exhaust gases but are in fact Chemtrails. The word "chemtrails" is a knock-off of the word "contrails." The term "chemtrail" was first introduced by a journalist, William Thomas, in 1997. People around the world have noticed that the weather conditions on the planet are changing dramatically. Also, they begin to notice the long lines left behind by the Airplanes. While there are many agendas associated with these malicious programs, the evidence is now abundant evidence that geoengineering can be used to control the weather. How long have chemtrails been going on? The chemtrail story was first told around 1997. In documentary films like: Why in the World are They Spraying, you will learn how aerosols sprayed into the sky are used in conjunction with other technologies to control the weather. If you talk in the rest of the world about airplanes that spray chemicals to change the weather, for sure they will think you are crazy, but in Countries like Thailand are real and on TV. Thai Pilots spray for the good of the nation, as Thai TV supports (Cloud Seeding). They do that to create rain so they can help the farmers. Is that the proof that chemtrails are real?

Cloud Seeding Chemtrails:

Cloud seeding started in 1946. Its A form of weather modification, usually by dropping suitable particles into clouds. Some people fear that weather modification could be used as a weapon to create natural disasters.

Is Cloud Seeding Harmful?

How much do we know about the environment? Should we be playing God and creating technology like cloud seeding? Are we able to accurately predict the effects? Can cloud seeding cause rain suppression, flooding, tornadoes, and silver iodide toxicity? On 16 August 1952, the UK government seeded the clouds and caused a terrible flood (Operation Cumulus project). Conspiracy theorists speculate that Project Cumulus contributed to the conditions that caused this flood, but the evidence was never found.

What Chemicals are Involved in Cloud Seeding?

Ice-forming (glaciogenic) and water-attracting (hygroscopic), compressed liquid propane and carbon dioxide, silver iodide (AgI), dry ice, salt, urea, and ammonium nitrate.

Is it Safe for Human, Animal and Plant Populations?

Carbon dioxide is mildly narcotic and toxic to the heart. Can cause diminished contractile force, increased blood pressure, pulse rate, reduced hearing, dizziness, confusion, and difficulty in breathing. The harmful effects of silver iodide are really dangerous. Intense exposure to silver iodide can cause temporary incapacitation.

Medical Internet and Search Engines Algorithms:
There are numerous dangers if you opt to self-diagnose using the internet. Pharmaceutical companies and dangerous Health websites sometimes spread ideas that can lead in the wrong direction and as a result, we get more stress and anxiety! The more stressed we are the easier we get symptoms that may not exist. It's so easy to trust search engine results when we're feeling not well. It is in human nature to assume the worst rather than the best. That is very true when it comes to mental illnesses, which often have overlapping symptoms. Just remember not all health sites are created equally and it's hard to know which one to trust. Internet health information can be your best friend or your worst enemy. Are most of these health websites coming first on the web search results because of the quality content or are there for a reason? Example: You search for Asthma attack symptoms and you get results for panic attacks. Then you read about the symptoms and you get more and more stress because it's almost the same. So, in the end, you think that maybe it's a panic disorder and not asthma. Of course, asthma can also cause dizziness palpitations, and shortness of breath! Unfortunately, most psychiatric websites do not explain that it is normal to have anxiety attacks when there is a reason, or when we have side effects from medications, and when we consume too much caffeine and that many diseases can mimic the symptoms of anxiety, such as GERD, asthma, diabetes, hypertension and so on.

Google Medic Update:

On August 1, 2018, a year before COVID 19 a new Google algorithm update takes place with the nicknamed "Medic". A large number of websites were affected by this Google core algorithm update. Sixty percent were medical and wellness websites. fitness niches, natural treatments niches, nutrition niches, and so on. Of course, some of the high domain authority pharmaceutical websites received a little extra boost in rankings. Google still informs the public that this is a global update that involves all searches and not only health sites, but everyone knows that this algorithm hit the medical/health niche the hardest. Some owners of health-related websites comment that this update took 50% of the traffic away almost overnight. Some others said that this is because Google focuses on domain 'trust' about health and that's why Google hit hard only on medical websites that don't toe the big pharma. Even trustable websites like dr Axe went down. Google also said that there is nothing you can do to fix your websites. Does that make sense? Now, many webmasters wonder who Google is, to tell if a website is good for health or has good medical advice, and with what criteria? People look on the internet for alternative health websites or natural remedies just because they don't trust doctors and pharmaceutical companies. So, what's the point of the medic algorithm?

FITNESS SECRETS, ADVENTURES AND SPORTS:

Fitness and nutrition, exercise tips. Sports include all forms of competitive physical activity. Any physical activity that improves or maintains physical fitness, overall health, and wellness is considered exercise. Physical fitness is one of the cornerstones of a happy, healthy life.

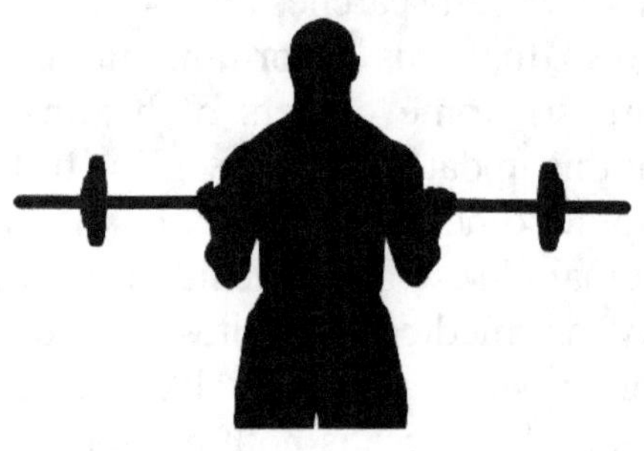

Creatine for Muscle Recovery and Fat Loss:

Creatine is three amino acids: arginine, glycine, and methionine. It's made primarily in the kidneys and completed in the liver. Creatine it's found in red meat, fish, dairy, and eggs. I was very skeptical if I needed to take a creatine supplement or not, but after a lot of research, I understood that is a supplement with not so many side effects and with a lot of benefits. Of course, it's better to take creatine from food sources and not from supplements, but I wanted to make an experiment and see how it will work with my body. After all, creatine supplements are made from organic molecules. So I decided to give it a shot because it is beneficial to muscle recovery, fat loss (particularly creatine HCL), powerlifting, and longevity. So, I chose to take creatine HCL because HCL has fewer side effects, does not require a loading phase, takes lower doses, and feels less bloating. Another benefit of creatine HCL is that is absorbed by the intestines about 60% better than creatine monohydrate.

The Results of Creatine HCL:

Now I understand why creatine is one of the best-selling supplements in bodybuilding communities. This supplement is not a steroid but works. It is a phenomenon for boosting your energy levels (Creatine Phosphate Stores and ATP). In short, creatine supplementation has been shown to improve maximal power and strength by up to 15%.

Creatine for Muscle Recovery:

Many so-called experts will tell you that creatine does not reduce muscle damage and does not help with muscle recovery, fortunately, they are wrong. Creatine supports protein synthesis, and as a result, your muscles recover faster from a workout. Studies have shown that creatine supplementation reduces muscle damage and inflammation. Another study proves that Creatine supplementation enhances muscle force recovery after eccentrically-induced muscle damage in healthy individuals.

Creatine Only on Workout Days?

You will not get the same benefits as taking it every day, but a new study suggests that muscle saturation is maintainable even if you don't take creatine every day. In my opinion, it's better to take creatine (after your 3-week load phase) only on your lifting days, and that's not forever. Use it just to build muscle for some time and then quit supplements and try to take creatine from natural sources. Why? Because the human body is lazy and instead of producing creatine is using the supplement. That's bad news as our body slows down the Creatine production.

Creatine HCL and Fat Loss:

All forms of creatine can help you with fat loss, as they will increase anaerobic power and cardio performance. So the harder you work out, the more calories you going to burn. I wrote creatine HCL for a reason. According to a new study, only Creatine HCl induced changes in body composition in recreational weightlifters. After the study, the results showed that fat mass was significantly decreased in HCl-1 groups.

Is Dirty Bulking a Good Idea?

Clean bulking is the best, that's for sure, even though, I intend to combine some healthy foods with fast food and sweets for 25 days before hitting the gym, working out hard, and analyzing the results. Then finally, I will try to get lean again and see if I gain more muscles. After all, whatever we are eating, junk food or healthy food, the calories are calories, right? Not really, healthy calories are better as you store less fat. Eating for pleasure is a form of wellness because hedonism has numerous health advantages. So, from time to time, eating bad food, such as pizza, is not a bad idea. But if you overdo it, you will become unhealthy and you will get sick. The bad news about this experiment is that if you eat crap for more than two weeks, you will feel bad about yourself and gain a lot of weight for no reason. Some argue that dirty bulking is a waste of time because your body will convert the rest of the food you don't need into fat, and I will agree to some extent. So, that's the reason I said before to don't overdo it. Dirty bulking has more benefits than just pleasure. You get more energy and stamina at the gym and by lifting heavier weights you gain bigger muscles.

Conclusion: In my opinion, dirty bulking is good for two weeks once a year, for pleasure, and rest. Now, as I previously stated, be dirty, but also eat some healthy foods if you don't want to store too much fat.

Gym Myths:

There are so many Gym myths and advice out there that can slow down your progress. One thing to keep in mind is that fitness science is changing all the time, one study shows something and the next study proves it wrong. So, always keep something if it works for you. Here are the top misleading fitness tips:

A Low Carb Diet for Long Time:

Yes, a low-carb diet is working, but that's not the only way to burn fat. The reason that a low-carb diet is the most famous way to burn fat is that people are very impressed by the quick results of a low-carb diet in the beginning. Now the reality is that we need healthy carbs, so I do not recommend a low-carb diet for a long time. Carbs are pure energy and you need them if you want to be strong at the gym. Instead, you can get have a low-calorie diet with all macronutrients. Carbs, Fat and Protein.

Cardio Eat your Muscles:

In reality, if you add cardio into your workout plan is the key to bigger muscles. Intense cardio sessions can improve your muscles' ability to neutralize lactic acid. For sure if you train like a marathon runner you will lose muscles, but if you do some HIIT exercises or some slow cardio, you will have more benefits. Aerobic and resistance training are completely compatible.

Six Pack are Made in Kitchen:

For sure nutrition is one of the most important factors for a six-pack, and yes, what you eat is more important than how much you exercise if you want to see your abdominal muscles. But just remember, abs are like any other muscle of your body. If you want to see some quick results, and if you want to have more shape and definition, then for sure you need to do crunches and situps.

Protein Should be Consumed Within 30 Minutes After a Workout:

I think we all know that behind this myth are the protein shake companies. First, never ignore real food for a protein shake. I see many guys finish Gym and look for a protein shake even if there are so many restaurants around. A recent study showed that the post-workout window is much bigger than the 30 minutes window. So don't overthink it. You have a 4 hours window and matters more what you will eat the rest of the day.

You can't Gain Muscle After 40:

That's a lie. For sure it will be harder and you will need some help if you have hormonal deficiencies, but if you look for testosterone, don't forget to do it the natural way. There are plenty of natural or herbal testosterone boosters out there.

Eat Every 2-3 Hours for a Faster Metabolism:

This is definitely false and studies have shown this is not the case. There's no point in eating 8 meals a day if you don't want to. The need to eat every 2-3 hours to boost your metabolism is completely wrong as simply your body is not a computer. So how many times do I have to eat? The best way is to listen to your body's hunger. The only good about eating every 2-3 hours is if you want to split your protein into many meals.

You Can't Gain Muscle and Lose Fat at the Same Time:
You can definitely gain muscle and lose fat at the same time, but it will take longer to see the results. The only thing you will need is to cycle your carbs. carbohydrate cycling intake is the key to success.

I Need a Lot of Protein to Build Muscles:
Yes, you need protein but not a lot of protein. Too much protein is bad for your kidneys and lymphatic system. The total amount of protein needed is less than most people think. You need only 1-1.2 grams of protein per pound of body weight. Excess protein is stored as fat, so if you eat more than that, your body will convert protein into fat.

Jump Rope Health Benefits:

Jumping rope is one of the best cardio for fat loss and has a lot of benefits. Many famous boxers or martial artists were big fans of jumping rope and that's for a reason, including Mike Tyson, Muhammad Ali, Chuck Norris, Bruce Lee, etc. There are multiple jump rope techniques like Crossovers, Single freestyle, Double Jumps, Single speed, High knees and so on. How many calories does rope jumping burn per minute? According to a What's Cooking America study, you can burn 130 calories in 10 minutes. But what about the health benefits?

Simplicity:
Some of the benefits of jumping rope are freedom and simplicity. You can take your Jumping rope almost everywhere.

Best Cardio for Fat Loss:
Better than running, jumping rope is the best calorie-burner, you can burn 130 calories in 10 minutes.

Stamina:
We all know that Jumping Rope helps you to build stamina and improves your aerobic capacity.

Best HIIT Cardio:
Without a doubt, Jump Rope is one of the best high-intensity exercises out there.

A Full-Body Exercise:
As is a full-body exercise, Rope jumping engages every muscle in your body.

Abs Muscles:
Rope Jumping is a dynamic core exercise and is a hard workout for your abs.

Is Good for your Heart:
Jumping has a lot of benefits for cardiovascular health, as it helps with blood pressure, reduces heart rate, and increases oxygen consumption.

Eliminates Stress:
Jumping rope benefits extend beyond your muscles, it stimulates your brain activity and releases endorphins, which reduces stress.

Finally, another great advantage of rope jumping is that you can do it before Weight Training (rather than using a treadmill), as you can burn more fat.

Mind Sports:

There are so many games called mind sports. Mind Sports are sports in which the objective is to test mental strength rather than physical strength. Some of them are board games, chess, card games, backgammon, billiard games (Pool/Snooker), darts, and video games. My favorite mind sports are chess, billiard games, and video games. I used to spend a lot of time playing chess and betting on pool games as a kid, but video games were where I spent the most time. Since I can't study every sport, I'll focus on one of my favorites: video games.

Positive and Negative Effects of Playing Videos Games:

What are the positive and negative effects of playing video games? How much virtual reality is too much? Everything has good and bad sides; therefore, the issue is how we use video games. As a child, I loved to play video games, but now that I'm older I started to realize more about the dangers of virtual reality. I still enjoy playing video games, but only when a new, excellent game is out, and I don't play for more than four hours per week. To play for an hour, four times per week is ideal in my opinion. Do not play video games with violent content or ones that include subliminal messages that could harm your subconscious mind. Below is a list of the advantages of playing video games, which are supported by studies.

The Positives of Playing Video Games:

Video Games Enhance Creativity:
Children who play video games tend to be more creative.

Video Games Help Relieve Pain:
Research revealed that playing video games can help to relieve pain.

Planning and Manage Limited Resources:
The player learns how to manage limited resources.

Accuracy:
Video games force kids to think quickly. According to a study, action games, help the player's brain to make faster decisions.

Video Games Help to Increase Memory:
Video games can help to improve memory.

Education:
Playing the right video games can help you educate.

Concentration and Focus:
According to study video games can help you concentrate and focus on one thing.

Maths and Solutions:
Video games with puzzles can help you to find solutions.

Games are everywhere today you can play games on your smartphone, television, or the Internet, but excessive gaming can affect negative your life.

The Negatives of Playing Video Games:

Addiction:
Video game addiction can be harmful to us and our children.

Increases Aggressive Behavior:
Video games that have violent scenarios may lead addicted players to be desensitized to violence.

Social Isolation:
Spending too much time playing games leads to loneliness and social isolation.

Negative Subconscious Mind:
Don't forget that the media-built characters. Subliminal hidden messages in some games affect negatively the subconscious mind.

Should you Eat Before Working out?

So, which is the best pre-workout food for fat loss? It's not an easy question. It all depends on your personal goals. There are numerous opinions on what is the best pre-workout food for fat loss. Is a perplexing subject because there are so many different experts who all have different and contrasting viewpoints. Unfortunately, most pre-workout meals are not good for fat loss. Wrong Pre-workout meals that are high glycemic and carbs will inhibit fat burning.

Fasting Before Exercise for Dramatic Loss of Fat:

Some research showed that intermittent fasting induces even stronger rejuvenating effects on cells and tissues. Intermittent fasting is not a diet, it is a diet system. "Eat, Fast, Live Longer," is a documentary on BBC with the Journalist Michael Mosley. Michael Mosley examined whether fasting helped people to live better and more. He found out after experiencing various forms of intermittent fasting, that the "5: 2" system, (which includes reducing your calorie intake by 25% for only two days a week) is the best. So, according to some researchers, intermittent fasting and exercise produce great results in fat loss.

Consume Healthy Carbs:

What you consume prior to working out has an impact on your performance. For example, if your goal is to lift weights at the gym, you will require fuel. Eating a light snack 45 to 60 minutes earlier is an excellent idea. This snack should also be nutritious and contain carbs, fats, and proteins. Some healthy options are full-fat yogurt with granola and your favorite fruit, protein-packed smoothies, oatmeal with almond milk, and so on.

Low Carb Diet and Sore Muscles:

Everybody knows that Low-Carb diets are good for health as you lose fat and you get lean muscles! But in my opinion, carbs are in nature for a reason. So, the real question for us when we are on low carbs is, what's the deal with a low-carb diet and sore muscles? I love fitness and in general a healthy lifestyle. So, I cut carbs to get a lean shredded body. As some experts advised me at the gym, fewer carbs lead to leaner muscles. So far so good. But, when I was younger, I had a motorbike accident and as a result of the titanium surgical plate that I have on my leg, I developed Piriformis syndrome. Piriformis muscle is one of the causes of sciatica. So, after a month of a low-carb diet, I felt a very strange pain in my left lower back. The pain got worse after the low-carb diet and over the next week, I felt very tired.

Ketosis Muscle Pain:

So, cutting out carbs can lead to fat loss, but with a risk. Our body stores carbs in the muscles in the form of glycogen together with fats that are used during exercise for energy. Low-Carb Diets can cause muscle aches, cramps, and pains. Leg cramps are very common when starting a low-carb diet and it is a side effect of loss of minerals (mostly magnesium). The solution here is to increase the intake of water and salt, take a supplement with magnesium if needed, and in the end increase your healthy carbohydrate intake. Don't forget that moderation is the key to a lean muscular body. Eating too much protein can also seriously harm your kidneys. Balance your diet as your body needs healthy carbohydrates to break down the proteins you consume. Here are some other keto-flu symptoms: nausea, vomiting, headache, sleeplessness, constipation, dizziness, and fatigue during the workout.

Protein and BCAA Supplements:

Peeople starting at the gym, have so many questions about protein Supplements. Here are some fundamental questions: Can protein help me gain muscle? Protein and BCAA supplements: natural or synthetic? Should you consume a protein shake before or after working out? How soon after exercise should I consume protein? Let's start with the most important question:

Are Proteins and BCAA Organic Natural Supplements?

Protein YES! Protein is derived from many different food sources like Rice Egg, Milk, Soy, Hemp, Pea, and so on. Most manufacturers also fortify their products with minerals, amino acids, vitamins, greens, grains, additional fats, fiber, and so on. Egg-based protein supplements are around since the 1950s and Whey protein is actually a byproduct of making cheese. Now about BCAA are not all companies good and natural. Not all BCAAs are created equal. There are many ways to produce amino acids and unfortunately, the most common method is a harsh acid extraction of animal products like duck feathers and human hair. The best method for the production of amino acids is through the fermentation of cultures in a pharmaceutical lab. So, when you buy BCAAs, try to buy fermented natural BCAAs. Fermentation or bioconversion using enzymes.

Do I Need Protein and BCAA Supplements?

Yes and no. The most important thing to remember here is that you should consume your protein within two to four hours after your workout. So, whether you are hungry or not, you must consume a post-workout meal, and because it is difficult to cook something, many people prefer to drink a protein shake.

Drink Protein Before or After a Workout?

According to Dr. Jeff Volek (a Famous dietitian-scientist) is better if you split your protein supplement intake in two when training: Half protein supplement 30 minutes before your workout and the other half within 30 minutes after your workout.

Swimming Workout:

S wimming is one of the best aerobic exercises with also a very low risk of injury. It's one of the few exercises which train nearly all muscle groups in the entire body, but different swimming strokes exercise better in different muscle groups. Water is nearly 800 times denser than air, so workout inside water makes you stronger. Swimming can give you strength, flexibility, and stamina and help you lose weight. In this chapter, we will learn which muscles are used during the various swimming strokes.

Muscles Used in Front Crawl Stroke - Freestyle:

The front crawl is the most known swimming stroke and is the most popular stroke in freestyle races, but what muscles are used in the front crawl Stroke? The primary muscles used in front crawl stroke are the shoulders, abdominal, leg, and back muscles.

Muscles Used in Breaststroke:

The breaststroke style is one of the most popular swimming strokes. The swimmer uses arms and legs synchronously. The muscles used are about the same for breaststroke, butterfly, and freestyle. The brachioradialis muscles in the arms, the glutes, and the chest and upper back muscles are the main muscles used in the breaststroke.

Muscles Used in Backstroke:

Backstroke is one of the best exercises for back pain and it improves your posture. It's also the only stroke that helps you so much with abdominal core muscles. The primary muscles used in the Backstroke are the muscles of your back, your legs, your arms, and shoulders, and finally, your abdominal core muscles.

Muscles Used in Butterfly Stroke:

It's one of the most recent strokes and was developed in the 1950s. The butterfly stroke is the second fastest stroke after freestyle. The primary muscles used in butterfly stroke are the biceps brachii and brachialis at the top of your upper arms, the pectoralis in your chest, and the latissimus dorsi in your back, drawing.

HIIT Swimming Workout:

High-Intensity Interval Training (HIIT) is one of the best cardio exercises today. It's the fastest, most efficient way to get in shape and burn more fat. High-intensity interval training is done when elevating your heart rate for a brief period, followed by resting for a given period. A perfect example is when running. Sprinting for one minute and then walking for two minutes is high-intensity interval training. Just remember HIIT training, wasn't meant to be done every day. There are many ways that you can do high-intensity interval training, but what about swimming? Can you do high-intensity interval training with swimming? Swimming is an incredible body workout. I love swimming and after a lot of research and questions, I found that you can do a HIIT workout with swimming.

Swimming is an excellent cardio and another important benefit is that pool water provides resistance while swimming, which makes our muscles work harder, as a result, swimming decreases your time in the gym and grows your muscles in less time!

Here is a Swimming HIIT Program:
100m warmup - freestyle at a slow pace
40m - sprint freestyle
80m - slow freestyle
Repeat with any swimming stroke you like (freestyle, backstroke, breaststroke, or butterfly) and add more meters if necessary.

Hatha Yoga Asanas:

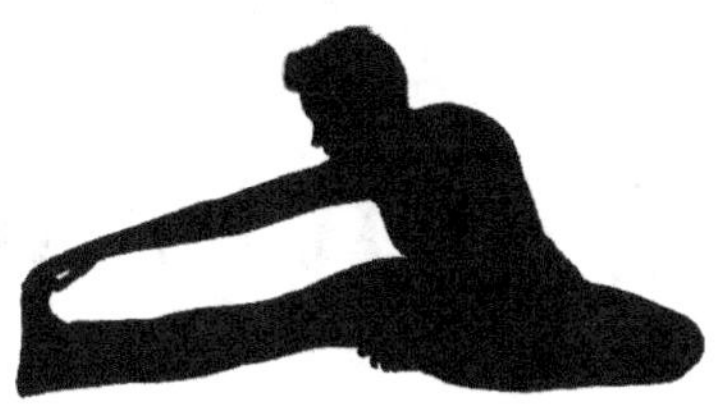

In India and Nepal, I learned the first steps of Yoga and meditation from experienced Yoga teachers and Monks. Today I still practice yoga Asanas, Pranayama, and Meditation techniques. Yogis always do yoga before meditating. Yoga improves flexibility and releases energy in the body. As a result, yoga helps the body to sit still for long periods while meditating. Hatha Yoga is my favorite as it is smoother for my bones. Asana means posture. Yoga asanas are extremely beneficial for our mental and physical well-being. Yoga is not just exercise. With asanas, you can manipulate the energy of your body in a certain direction. Hatha yoga techniques are useful for balancing the body and mind.

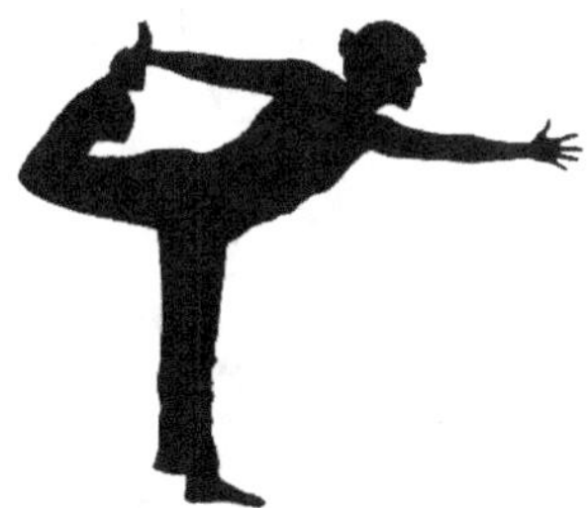

'Ha' represents the sun, and 'tha' the moon. With Hatha yoga, you can manipulate the positive and negative energies of your body. Just like in Ayurveda, the traditional Indian medicine, Asanas in yoga are utilized for controlling the five elements: earth, water, fire, air, and spirit.

ASANAS HEALTH BENEFITS

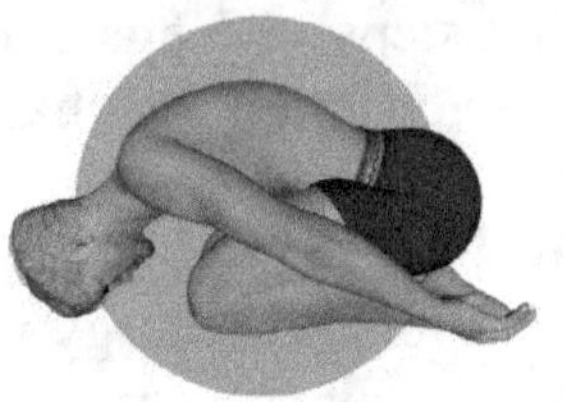

CHILD'S POSE

Child's pose can promote awareness and relaxation, regardless of your level of yoga experience. Also, your hip and back-supporting muscles can be stretched.

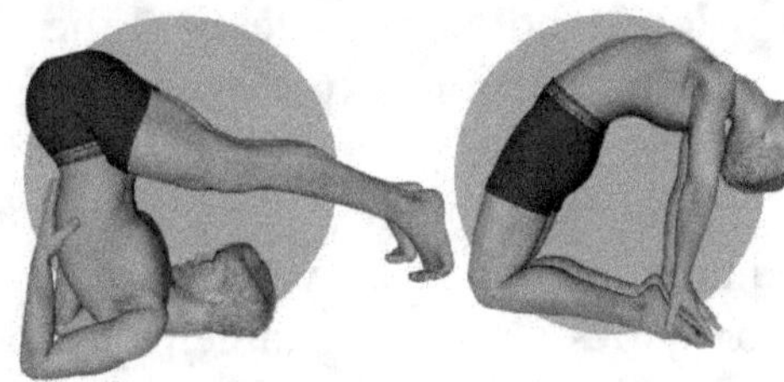

PLOW POSE

It reducing and releasing tension in your neck, shoulders, and back. Additionally, the position strengthens your legs, arms, and shoulders.

USTRASANA

Improves digestion. Stretches and strengthens the shoulders and back while opening up the hips and reducing thigh fat.

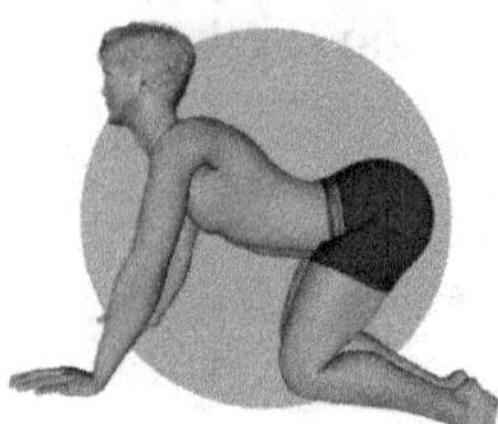

COW POSE

Cow pose helps to ease upper-body tension. In particular your back, shoulders, and neck. It massages the spine gently to improve mobility.

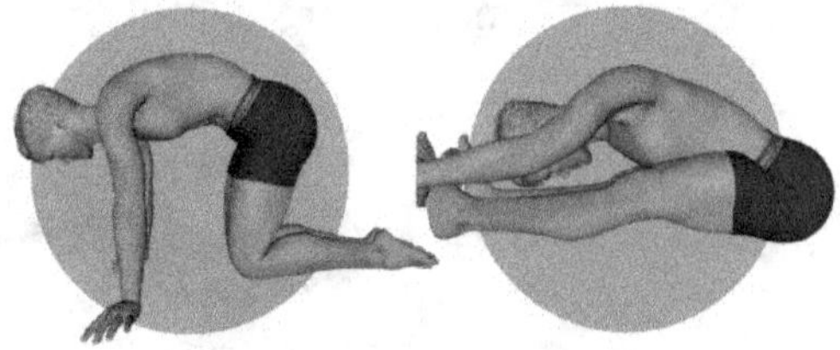

CAT POSE

This asana increases spinal fluid circulation and relieves stress from menstrual cramps, lower back pain, and sciatica.

SEATED FOLD POSE

The front fold pose stimulates the reproductive and urinary systems while calming the neurological system.

ASANAS HEALTH BENEFITS

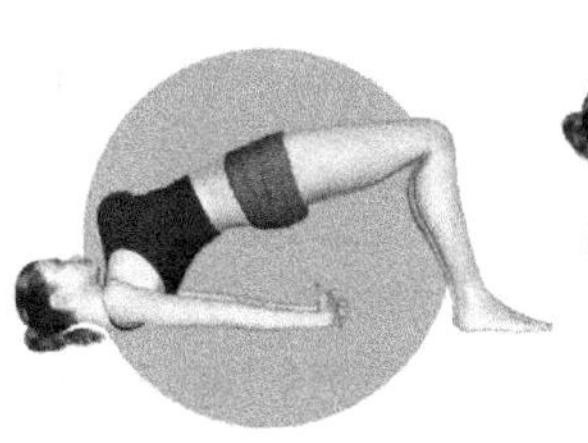

PURVOTTANASANA

Purvottanasana strengthens the body and promotes blood flow throughout it. Additionally, it thought to open the crown chakra as well as the solar plexus chakra.

BOAT POSE

The boat posture strengthens your arms and legs, especially your upper arms, as well as every part of your core.

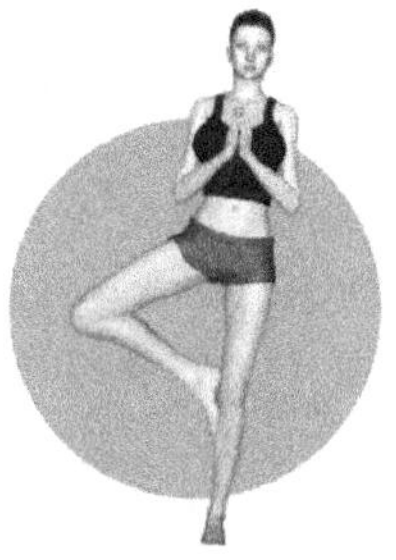

TREE POSE

Tree Pose is a balancing position that can boost confidence and make you feel rejuvenated. Additionally, it tones the core and legs.

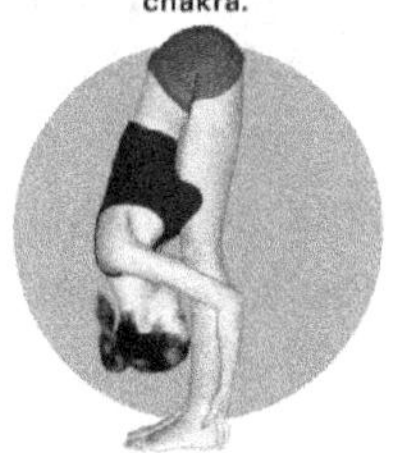
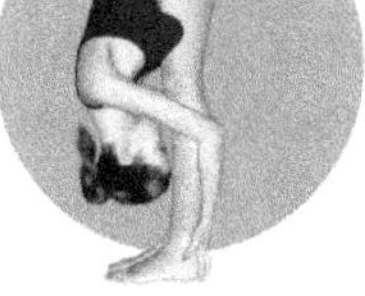

UTTANASANA

The forward fold posture improves digestion while stimulating the kidneys and liver. Decreases anxiety and blood pressure.

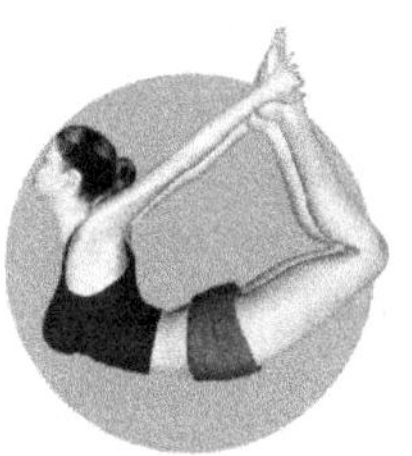
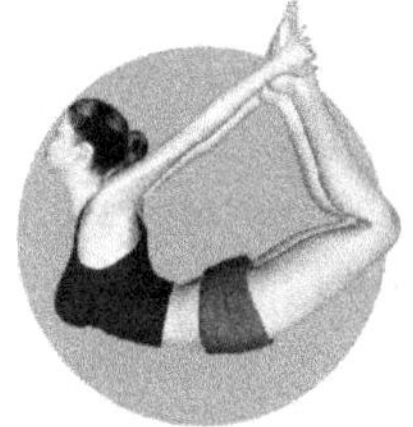

BOW POSE

Dhanurasana asana is particularly beneficial to the chest and back. It may also help in the muscle tone and strengthening of abdominal muscles.

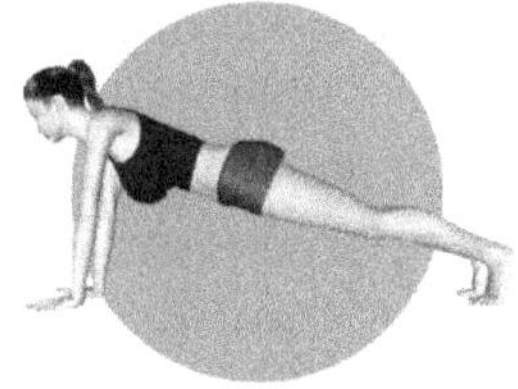

HIGH PLANK

High Plank is an excellent posture-improving pose because it strengthens a wide range of muscular and skeletal areas.

Sauna and Muscle Growth:

Sauna has a lot of benefits and nearly every health club has one, but is sauna good or bad for muscle growth? Can you use the sauna after a day at the gym? For sure if you use the sauna after a hard workout, it will help you to relieve sore muscles. Due to the hard kickboxing training, I have some muscle problems, and my physio suggested I use the sauna after working out. So, every time I go to the gym I end up in the sauna as it helps my muscles to relax and when muscles relax, are also growing. Muscle soreness always takes place after a workout, as tiny tears in your muscle fibers create micro-trauma. Heat therapy stimulates hormone production and can help release endorphins. In general, using a Sauna will help you to increase blood flow. Also, it will eliminate lactic acids and toxins released during exercise.

Can Sauna Raise Human Growth Hormone Levels?

Growth hormone (somatotropin) is a hormone that stimulates growth, and cell reproduction-regeneration in humans. According to a study from NCBU, HGH can increase muscle mass and reduce the amount of body fat. That means that saunas indeed will improve your workout performance. Another research showed that growth hormone levels increase from two to five times during sauna seasons. HGH is also the key to slowing the aging process.

Extreme Sports and Health:

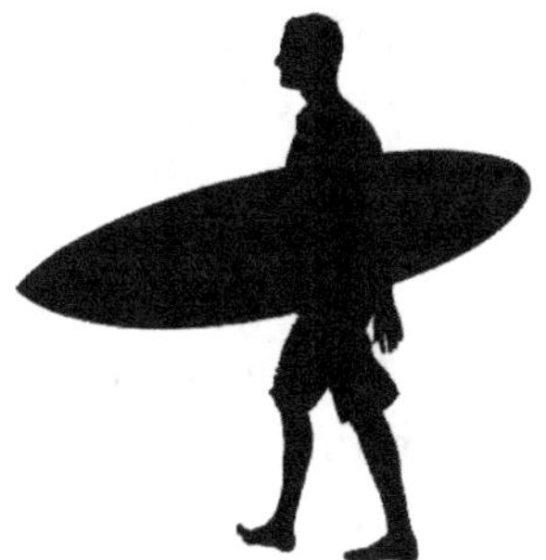

An extreme sport is a term for certain activities with a high level of danger. These activities often involve a high level of physical exertion, so are you ready to push yourself further than you ever thought? For me, the main reason that I like extreme sports is that you can become one with nature. If you do extreme sports carefully you can gain a lot of health benefits but don't forget that extreme sports are linked to 40,000 head and Neck injuries per year.

Extreme Sports List:

Air:
Jumping, Wingsuiting, Slacklining, Skydiving, Bungee Jumping, High-lining, Hang Gliding, Paragliding.

Earth:
Skateboarding, Mountain Boarding, Sandboarding, Caving, Motocross, Drifting, Aggressive Inline Skating, BMX and Mountain Biking, Absailing, Bouldering, Rock Climbing or free Climbing, Mountaineering, Parkour, Zorbing, Sand kiting.

Water:
Surfing, Bodyboarding, Cave diving, Wakeboarding, Waterskiing, Kitesurfing, Windsurfing, Kayaking, Paddle surfing, Cliff Jumping, Coasteering, Kneeboarding, snorkeling, Scuba Diving, White Water Rafting, skimboarding, Jet Skiing.

Snow and Ice:
snow skiing, Snowmobiling, Snowboarding, Ice Climbing, Snow Kiting.

Those are the main extreme sports, but many other extreme sports are not included in the list for example martial arts and many more. You will find more about the benefits of martial arts in my "Ancient and Traditional Healing Secrets Book Series."

Extreme Sports Benefits and Health Promotion:
Adventure sports play a leading role in the promotion of health, and despite the term "adrenaline junkie", extreme sports are healthy and can push you to your physical and mental limits.

Fun and Fitness:
Extreme sports will help in the pumping of pleasure-pumping chemicals. So, you can have a lot of fun, but you also exercise multiple muscle groups at once.

Win your Fears and get Self-Confidence:
A study found that participating in extreme sports, will actually give you a mental boost and give you self-Confidence.

Stress Relief and Sense of Reality:
Extreme athletes have lower anxiety and a higher sense of reality. Get new experiences and the opportunity to live life.

Humility:
With extreme sports, you understand that you are not immortal and as a result, you gain a sense of humility.

Increase your Balance:
It is no secret that dangerous extreme sports can help you increase your balance.

Burn Calories:
It keeps us extremely fit. Extreme sports are one of the best ways to burn calories.

Be One with Nature:
Extreme sports are outdoor activities that help us get in touch with nature.

Adrenaline Hormone and Dopamine:
There's a reason why extreme sports athletes are known as "adrenaline junkies." Adrenaline releases endorphins and neurotransmitters like dopamine, the chemical that makes you feel euphoric. Bardo's studies in the documentary Adrenaline Rush the Science of Risk showed that people who were high novelty seekers had lower levels of dopamine in their brains. So extreme sports participants are much better at handling stress.

Point Break Ozaki 8 List:

I'm a big fan of extreme sports and when I saw for the first time the movie Point Break (1991), with Patrick Swayze, Keanu Reeves, Gary Busey, and the Red-Hot Chili Peppers, I was fascinated. The absolute extreme sports movie. A gang of surfers against the system. The system that kills the human spirit. They robbed banks so they can do more extreme sports. I love the term adrenaline junkie and 24 years later, I saw the same title in the theaters: Point Break (2015). At the start, I thought it will be a remake of the old film, but I was wrong, the new movie is not just a copy of the old, it continues where the old movie left us. Although there share many similarities in the script, the new Point Break has even more ideas about the benefits of extreme sports. Extreme sports can make you feel one with nature. That's the main idea of that movie and I love it. The movie is not so much about surfing, like the old one. The new Point Break has even more extreme sports. The movie has to do with the top extreme sports worldwide - The Ozaki 8 list, but is this Ozaki 8 list real?

Is Ozaki 8 Real?

The first thing that I did when I finish watching the movie was to go online and research for the Ozaki 8 list, so I typed, is Ozaki 8 Real? What I have found is that the so-called Ozaki extreme sports Guru does not exist. What about the list, was a fiction or not? Well, Ozaki's list was fiction, until now. Now it's real, after the new Point Break movie. Nothing on the Ozaki list is impossible and if you do it you will have a whole new respect for nature and yourself. Ozaki 8 is a philosophy and way of living. So YES, Ozaki list it's real now. The idea is real, and so is the sports.

Ozaki 8 List:

Ozaki 8 Ordeals: Emerging Force, Birth of Sky, Awakening Earth, The Life of Water, Life of Wind, Life of Ice, Master of Six Lives, The act of Ultimate Trust

Ordeal 1 - Emerging Force - Rafting: LOCATION: In Ozaki list was at the Inga Rapids of the river Congo.

Ordeal 2 - Birth of Sky - Base Jumping: LOCATION: In Ozaki list was at MT Everest.

Ordeal 3 - Awakening Earth - Skydiving: LOCATION: In Ozaki list was at caves of shadows Mexico.

Ordeal 4 - Life of Water - Surfing: LOCATION: In Ozaki list was at the French Coast.

Ordeal 5 - Life of Wind - Wingsuit Flying: LOCATION: In Ozaki list was at Walenstadt Switzerland.

Ordeal 6 - Life of Ice - Snowboard: LOCATION: In Ozaki list was at Golden, British Columbia.

Ordeal 7 - Master of Six Lives - Climb: LOCATION: In Ozaki list was at angels falls Venezuela.

Ordeal 8 - Act of Ultimate Trust - Rope Jumping: LOCATION: In Ozaki list was at angels falls Venezuela and it was without the rope. Is like you put your life in nature's hands - Ultimate Trust. (Not Recommended) We add a Rope Jumping instant.

Theme Parks Health Benefits:

As a wellness seeker, I had to write about theme parks and their health benefits. There are several ways that a theme park can be good for your health. A Theme Park or an amusement park is a group of adventure attractions and entertainment attractions. I love theme parks. The first park that I visited was Disneyland in Paris and from that time, I became a big fan. My favorites are the water parks. For me is one of the safest ways to achieve some adrenaline, screams, and happiness. I can categorize these parks "in a way" into the extreme sports category. So, if you like fast extreme rides and adrenaline rush, here are some health benefits:

Burn calories while riding.
Relieves stress.
Improve your mood with fun and entertainment.
Provides a rush of adrenaline.
Overcome your fears.
Socialize.
It improves blood circulation.
You get a natural high.

Traveling Health Benefits:

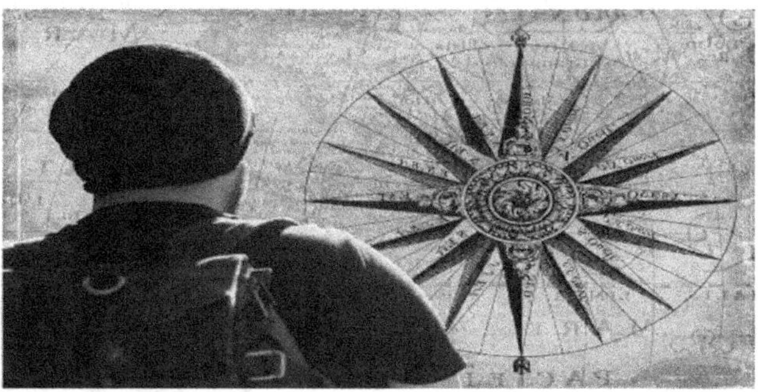

Traveling for me is one of the deepest forms of wellness and my work as a researcher will be incomplete if I don't explain my travel Philosophy. I've always been fascinated by traveling, meeting people from different cultures, trying new foods and ideas, but the most important thing for me was the intense experiences I was getting. Everyone wants to have a life full of memories after all. So, I was traveling around from a very small age and right now, I'm so glad that I did it. The first country I visited was Sweden. That times I didn't even know why I was traveling and why that was so important to me. Well, the travel instinct was in me, I just hadn't discovered it yet. Later on, it became clear that travel, exploration, and wellness were all part of the same philosophy path.

When I was 23, I created three very successful travel websites: the Explorers Journal, which was about exploration, travel, and archaeology secrets. The Travelers Meeting, which was a social media for those who were looking for a travel mate, and the Nighthawk Journeys which was about nightlife from around the world. In short, traveling became a way of living for me.

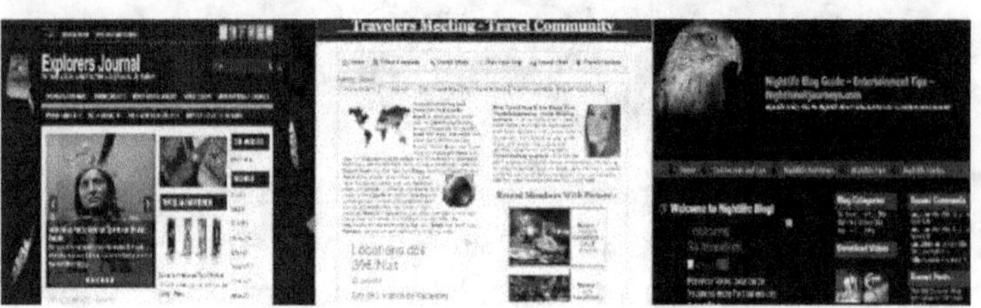

My most recent website is the wellness seeker which represents my understanding of the healing and travel connection firsthand. Let me now discuss the health advantages of traveling as I personally experienced them.

Travel Lowers Stress Levels:

Those who enjoy traveling are well aware that it is the best way to deal with stress and negative emotions. According to a study short vacation improves stress-levels and well-being.

Travel Improves Brain Creativity and Increase Mindfulness:

Travelling makes you smarter and broadens your perspectives. Different countries have different languages, different thinking different ways. In short, understanding other cultures opens your mind. Also, when you travel, you are so connected and focused that it is a form of mindfulness meditation.

Explore New Tastes and Flavors:

Different food has different health benefits. Nutrition is the most important thing for our health, we are what we eat after all. Every time you travel to another country, you will have the opportunity to try new herbs, spices, vegetables, fruits, and a variety of other nutritional products with delectable flavors you have never tasted before.

Get more Experiences:

Travelling creates lifetime memories that in my opinion those memories and experiences fill out our deepest levels of consciousness and help us to expand.

Travel Alone Boost Self-Confidence:

Increase your self-confidence with solo travel. I love to travel by myself. Solo travel helps us to research our inner selves and increase our awareness. Being responsible for yourself and enjoying your own company helps our personal growth.

Traveling Make you Social:
Get more comfortable talking to new people. Connect with the locals or other travellers and make new friends. Learn how to make friends out of strangers.

A Feeling of Wellness, Fullness and Wholeness:
It's true when traveling, you all have those moments of wellness, fullness, and wholeness. You became one with the world and the world one within you.

Adventure and Adrenaline Benefits:
Feel like an adventurer by riding an elephant or a camel in the desert, driving a jeep deep into the jungle, or participating in an extreme sport and experiencing the adrenaline rush. Adrenaline releases endorphins and neurotransmitters like dopamine, the chemical that makes you feel euphoric.

Travelling is a Good Exercise:
Traveling around, especially on backpacking promotes physical activity. Traveling around will make you more active and stronger, which is good for your heart.

Sites with Healing Properties:
Our planet offers many places with natural healing powers, and believe it or not science proves it with studies. Visiting healing sites with spiritual pathways gives you wellness with sacred healing properties.

Travel is Good for Longevity:
Traveling may hold the key to living a longer life. I believe that all of the other health benefits of traveling contribute to this. Many studies have found that traveling is one of the best ways to achieve longevity.

Traveling Lowers the Risk of Depression:
Do I need to cover that? We all know that travel boosts happiness, as I said above, travel is a stress-reducer.

It Helps us Escape from our Daily Routine:
Everybody needs life changes, and travel is the best way to escape from your daily routine. See the world, recharge your batteries, and build your experiences.

Why do Humans Need to Explore?
We all love adventure movies like Indiana Jones or games like the Tomb Raider and Uncharted, but why? Why do we love those kinds of movies, books, or games? I believe this is primarily due to the fact that people enjoy exploring, particularly ancient secrets from the past. For instance, while visiting Greece, you may enjoy the beaches and the delectable cuisine, but if you skip visiting one of the several historic archaeological sites, such as the Acropolis, your trip would be incomplete. The same goes for almost any other country like Cambodia, Egypt, China, Peru, Mexico, Thailand, etc. We are all fascinated so much about ancient secrets, scripts, ruins, books, and in general, knowledge from the past. The ancients knew so many secrets about longevity, medicine, and the afterlife, they had ancient technology and they were surrounded by mysticism. In ancient times everything was spiritual, the dances, the architecture, the ceremonies, etc.

So, the need for wellbeing is the primary driver behind humans' need for travel and our shared love of those kinds of explorations. Many secrets were discovered by our ancestors, and we all want to know what they were. While modern science and technology have taken much of this ancient knowledge from us. We want to take back what belongs to us. But isn't this just about the ancient secrets? What about sea exploration, space exploration, or any other type of exploration? Humans seeking answers about who we are and where we came from. What are the reactions of other creatures? Are we the only ones in the Universe? In short, humans are seeking answers and knowledge, and perhaps other life forms will provide solutions to our common diseases. Exploration has provided a lot of benefits to our society for centuries. We want to improve, to achieve perfection in our soul, mind, and body.

Our wonderful journey has come to an end, but our healing development continues. Health is everything and knowledge of health is crucial.

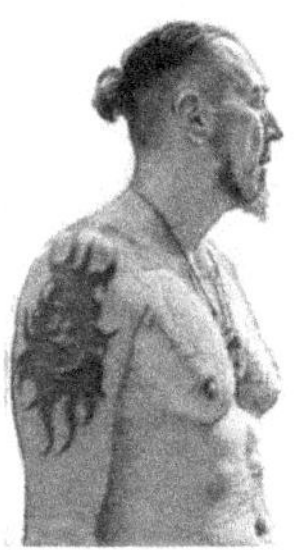

I hope you'll be inspired and make some life changes. Improve your quality of life through regular physical exercise, healthy nutrition and positive state of mind.

www.ingramcontent.com/pod-product-compliance
Lightning Source LLC
Chambersburg PA
CBHW061621250726

48659CB00004B/1033